THE SIMPLE 3-WEEK PLAN
FOR MORE ENERGY, BETTER SLEEP
& SURPRISINGLY EASY WEIGHT LOSS!

SUGAR FREE

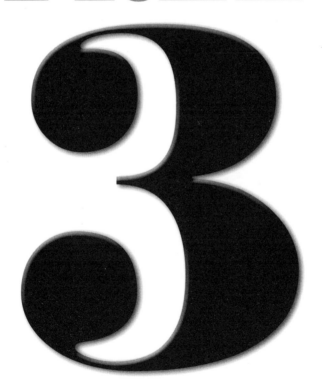

MICHELE PROMAULAYKO

FORMER EDITOR-IN-CHIEF of *WOMEN'S HEALTH* and *COSMOPOLITAN*

This book is intended as a general reference volume only, not as any form of medical treatment or advice. The information given here is designed to help you make informed decisions about your health and wellness. It is not provided or intended as any form of a medical diagnosis or plan, or a substitute for any treatment that may have been prescribed by your doctor. If you have any unique medical issues or conditions, or otherwise suspect that you may have a medical issue or sensitivity, please first consult with a medical provider before starting this or any other nutrition program to discuss your specific needs.

Creative Direction and Book Design: J. Heroun

Library of Congress Cataloging-in-Publication Data

Name: Promaulayko, Michele, author.

Title: SUGAR FREE 3 : THE SIMPLE 3-WEEK PLAN FOR MORE ENERGY, BETTER SLEEP & SURPRISINGLY EASY WEIGHT LOSS! / MICHELE PROMAULAYKO

New York, NY
ISBN-10: 1940358418
ISBN-13: 978-1940358413

Published by Openfit LLC
ɔpenfit.

www.openfit.com

Distributed to the book trade by Galvanized Media and Simon & Schuster

DEDICATION

TO ANYONE WHO HAS EVER HAS BEEN TRAPPED IN A
BAD RELATIONSHIP WITH SUGAR, HERE'S TO BREAKING UP—
FOR GOOD! FREEDOM TASTES SO MUCH BETTER.

CONTENTS

FOREWORD

By David Zinczenko,
Founder and Author of *Eat This, Not That!*

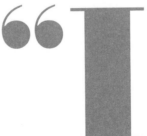"I JUST CAN'T LOSE WEIGHT!"

As the author of more than 20 health and wellness bestsellers, including *The Abs Diet* and *Eat This, Not That!*—and the onetime Editorial Director of *Men's Health* and *Men's Fitness*—I hear that exasperated claim all the time. Here's how I respond: There's no better or healthier way to lose weight—and keep it off—than to give up added sugars.

The trick is knowing how.

In **Sugar Free 3**, Michele Promaulayko tells you *exactly* how. First she unmasks the true culprit behind excess weight and poor health—sugar, specifically added sugars and their evil twins, refined carbs and artificial sweeteners—which food manufacturers sneakily slip into almost everything we eat, from bread to cold cuts to yogurt, peanut butter, and pizza. She exposes the dangers of a high-sugar diet and, more important, teaches you how to replace it with satisfying, hunger-reducing foods that put you on the path to a much healthier life.

You have the perfect guide in Michele, who has been at the forefront of the latest health and wellness research for over a decade and knows every expert worth knowing. Back when I was the Editorial Director of *Men's Health*, *Women's Health*, and *Prevention*—three of the leading magazines about healthy living—I hand-picked her to be the Editor-in-Chief of *Women's Health* after her editorial test blew me away. Candidates were meant to submit a few ideas. Michele submitted an entire magazine. And then she led the brand on a blockbuster run, building a community of readers who trusted her reporting because it worked. (She then did the same at Yahoo! Health and *Cosmopolitan*.)

I saw up close her dedication and talent for finding the best experts and ferreting out the soundest advice—and that's what **Sugar Free 3** is. It's the result of Michele interviewing thought-leaders like nutritionist Keri Glassman, health journalist Max Lugavere, movement expert Lauren Roxburgh, and dermatologist Dr. Whitney Bowe. She's developed a plan that's easy, effective, and works for everyone.

They contributed because they know how detrimental added sugar is, and they all trust Michele to deliver that message because she doesn't just talk the talk—she walks the walk (and then goes to a barre class afterward). Yet despite her commitment to a healthy lifestyle, Michele's had her own struggles with sugar, and inside you'll learn how she's loosened sugar's vice grip with the help of **Sugar Free 3**.

But don't just take it from her—or me. The very first people to try the program experienced more energy, better sleep, improved moods, fewer cravings, increased awareness in food choices and, of course, weight loss; 5 pounds, 10 pounds, 15 pounds and some even more in just 3 weeks. Here are a few of their success stories:

"My tummy is smaller and my clothes fit better. It's great for kicking off your weight loss journey."

—AMBER J.

"I feel so different than I did three weeks ago. I have so much more energy and mental strength. I feel much more confident about nutrition and health now. After realizing the results of the new lifestyle I am 100% ready to keep it going."

—MARIO C.

"My appetite has decreased. I am not as hungry all the time and I get full quicker. What I loved best about the program was all of the new things I learned, and I really like all the support from the group. It was really good to know I wasn't the only one with questions and to know I wasn't alone."

—JUDY G.

"I never paid attention to what I consumed or how much. But I have a lot more control now because I know how harmful sugar is to my body. In the last three weeks, I have seen many physical changes, such as weight loss all over my body down to my feet!"

—COURTNEE S.

Read on to discover how they transformed their relationship with sugar—and how you can, too.

To your good health,
Dave Zinczenko

INTRODUCTION

You *Can* Go Sugar Free. It Worked For Me!

By Simply Cleaning Up Your Diet
You Will Feel Better Than Ever Before

CONGRATULATIONS on taking a big step toward boosting your health and well-being. I'm so glad you're here. This book is not a diet. It's not a detox. It's not a cleanse. And it won't instruct you to do nutty things. **Sugar Free 3** works (and it works fast) because it's an easy and effective way to help you kick sugar, reset your body, and feel totally amazing! And just about everyone could benefit from consuming less sugar, me included.

As the former editor-in-chief of *Women's Health* and *Cosmopolitan*, I spent many years researching and writing about health, nutrition, and fitness—both fun trends and serious conditions. To be an editor, you need to be endlessly curious, but also pretty skeptical, because a major aspect of the job is sifting through the glut of information out there to determine what qualifies as the absolute best advice to share with readers.

Before starting my magazine career, I was active, but I wasn't necessarily healthy. I worked out and played sports, but my eating and sleeping habits were all over the map. And yeah, I did a fair bit of partying. I mean, I was a young editor grinding it out in New York City—it comes with the territory! I got invited to glam parties and star-studded premieres and a lot of other excessive soirees. It was fun as hell, but not awesome for keeping my health in check. And when the novelty of going out every night wore off, and I began to delve deeper into health topics, I developed a real passion for wellness. I also discovered just how badly Americans need help figuring out how to take better care of themselves. We're a nation obsessed with looking good, and yet statistics—or even a cursory glance around a grocery store—prove that we struggle with health and weight management. Our social media feeds and news channels are filled with posts about the latest silver-bullet solution—a cleanse, a fast, a miracle green juice, not to mention the hype around popular diets, such as paleo and keto, that cut out whole categories of food. And still, obesity rates rise. No doubt those kinds of plans work for some people, but they never worked for me, because they are just too restrictive and regimented. And I'm not alone in feeling that way, am I right?

Luckily, this book isn't about following a fad or a narrow list of allowable foods (grapefruit for breakfast, lunch, and dinner—I'll pass). Instead, I'm here to talk about how giving up added sugars for three short weeks can help change your life—and why I devised **Sugar Free 3** to help you do just that.

A Real Plan for Real People

For most of the year, I eat healthfully, exercise regularly, and work hard to look my best. (I'm not the young, survive-on-fumes editor I used to be!) But there are certain times throughout the year when the balance I normally achieve goes completely off the rails. Summer is one of those times because when the sun comes out, so does the sauvignon blanc...and the rosé...and a few nice chilled reds. I admit it—I'm a wino. Or, more accurately, a wine lover. When I plan vacations, I gravitate to places that are known to be top wine regions—France, Italy, Greece, Argentina, California—because to me, eating and drinking are huge and pleasurable parts of the holiday experience.

And who am I kidding—if they had gummy bear vineyards, I'd visit them, too! Second confession: I am a candy monster. I make no apologies for loving the sweet stuff—specifically, sour gummies and licorice. Yum! There is a certain Swedish shop called Sockerbit in downtown NYC that I find hard to walk past without filling up a bag of sugary, salty (great combo, by the way), chewy candies. Most of my friends have been dragged in by me on at least one occasion.

Listen, there's nothing wrong with a conscious indulgence here and there. But by the end of August, I am up to my eyeballs in dry white wine and pistachio ice cream cones (my other sweet vice) and feeling kinda crappy. That's when I know it's time for a sugar reboot. And this year, rather than trying to do penance by praying nobody invites me to happy hour, I wanted concrete, well-thought-through guidelines. I'm smart and experienced enough to know that recalibrating takes more than a torturous weekend cleanse. While I wanted to make some lifestyle changes, I wasn't looking for a forbidding forever plan. I just needed to rein it in. Shockingly, I couldn't find anything to *realistically* help me do it. So I decided to create something for myself—and for you.

I turned to some of the most respected wellness experts in the country to help me, people that I have used as resources in the magazines I've edited—and many of whom I now consider close friends. And we did it. **Sugar Free 3** will help you kick sugar safely and effectively, and and it's easier than you could ever imagine. You'll eliminate added sugars, refined carbs, and artificial sweeteners for just three weeks—and I'll show you exactly what to eat and what to avoid, step by step. And it doesn't matter how busy you are or what your lifestyle is, we've thought of everything to help you succeed. Even if, like me, you don't feel lousy on the regular, you will be mind-blown by how much *better* you feel when you ditch the unnecessary sugar. My skin looked glowier, I slept much more soundly, my digestion improved, and I had bonus energy, which helped power everything else I like and need to do, from exercising to tackling work projects. You, too, can experience these fantastic outcomes and more on **Sugar Free 3**. And I promise, you won't have to do anything extreme. You won't have to starve yourself or cut out all carbs. The goal isn't to become some "super clean" eater for life. You're going to eat whole, delicious food that will keep you satiated. The greatest part: You don't have to count calories or eat tiny portions.

It's a real plan for real people. But you don't need to take my word for it. People like Joslyn B., a marketing manager, and Courtnee S., a Head Start teacher, and Judy G., a stay-at-home mom, and the other test panelists tried **Sugar Free 3** and reported back having:

◆ *Healthier-looking skin*

◆ *Better quality sleep*

◆ *Fewer sweet cravings*

◆ *Stronger willpower*

◆ *Easier weight loss*

At the end of it, in addition to the benefits I've already listed, I lost six pounds—enough to help me comfortably fit back into my favorite jeans and feel like myself again. But what was most exciting is that for the first time in a long time I felt in control of my sugar cravings and consumption. And I began to approach my eating and drinking in a new, more informed way.

We All Have Our "Thing"

What's your thing? I mean, when it comes to sugar—what's the one thing you can't resist? Is it warm molten chocolate cake or a hot slice of apple pie with ice cream melting into the gooey center? Maybe it's gulping a fizzy, ice-cold soda on a hot summer day, or sipping a venti Frappuccino (extra whipped cream!) on the way to work, or downing a not-so-nutritious energy drink to keep you going past the three o'clock slump.

Sugar has been a "thing" for many of us since childhood. Growing up in a single-parent household, I had a pantry filled with Fruity Pebbles, Cocoa Puffs, and my fave, Lucky Charms ("They're magically delicious!"). Turns out, at the end of the rainbow pictured on the box was a vat of sugar, not a pot of gold. Our "health food" was Fig Newtons. Our "milk" was Yoo-hoo, the sugartastic chocolate beverage. Telling you this is not to diss my mom in any way. She was doing the best she could, and these kinds of foods were what lined—and still line—grocery store shelves. She didn't have the health knowledge I have now, so she wasn't aware of just how detrimental and habit-forming consuming all of that sugar was.

And it's not like I spent my youth riding the couch with my hand shoved into a cookie jar. I played soccer from third grade through high school. I dated a guy who was into fitness and supplements before it was popular, and who got me curious about nutrition. I also ate "fat-free" when that was all the rage in the '90s, thinking I was doing a good thing. What I didn't do was connect sugar with weight gain, or any other undesirable effects. Why would I? I wasn't overweight, per se. But I wasn't my ideal weight. My body composition was off: I was soft and puffy, not dense—my muscles were hiding under a mushy layer. I wasn't sick or lethargic, but I wished I had more energy, more focus.

These feelings continued into adulthood.

As an ambitious editor climbing the ladder of the magazine industry in New York City, I'd do cardio classes, indoor cycling, and floor exercises with ankle and wrist weights. But I'd start most mornings by eating a bagel the size of my head for breakfast (hey, it's fat free!) and end the evening with a takeout dinner of Thai food or pizza. By day, I was writing about fashion, beauty, and boys. By night, I was eating Snackwells by the sleeve. Anyone remember those?

When my income increased, so did the size of my kitchen—and my meals. Public relations companies plied me and my staff with sweets they'd send so that we'd pay attention to their products (it worked!). Every week there was a co-worker's birthday or anniversary to celebrate... with cake; offices, in general, tend to be littered with candy, chocolate, and baked goods. Movie premieres, book launches, and parties always had complimentary sweets, too—with cupcakes so small, it was easy to pop one (or five) in my mouth between glasses of champagne.

Looking at photos of myself from back then, I was a good 10 pounds heavier than I am today, with blotchy skin and tired eyes. It wasn't until I became the editor-in-chief of *Women's Health* magazine that it really hit me: I'd always worked out, but I was eating far more calories than I was burning. After all, you can't out-exercise a bad diet because it's way easier to take in empty calories than it is to burn them off.

The same is likely true for you. Even if you aren't into candy or ice cream, it's probable that you eat too many refined carbs or artificial sweeteners. The scary thing about sugar—which will be illuminated in this program—is that it hides in foods you may not think are sweet or "unhealthy," like spaghetti sauce, ketchup, bread, crackers, salad dressings, and yogurt—to name a few of the sneaky sources.

It's just about everywhere.

As a result, the average American consumes nearly 152 pounds of sugar annually—almost 30 pounds more than we did in 1970. That's almost 44 teaspoons daily, or three pounds a week! Many of these sugars are classified as "added sugars"—that is, sugars that are added to foods when they are processed or prepared. The American Heart Association recommends that men consume no more than 150 calories in added sugars daily, and women 100. But most of us are eating more than twice that amount—men are getting 335 calories in added sugar, and women 239—every single day! Eating so much sugar significantly raises your risk of life-shortening obesity, diabetes, and cardiovascular disease: A study in *JAMA Internal Medicine* found that people who exceeded the recommended daily limit of sugar increased their risk of death due to heart disease by at least 30 percent.

Artificial sweeteners, which are touted as the healthier alternative, come with a laundry list of potential health issues, including—believe it or not—weight gain. Yes, that diet soda you think is helping you stay slim may be making you fatter.

It's Not Your Fault

Our sweet teeth are nothing new. Nor are they totally our fault. In fact, humankind's attraction to sugar is part of how we survived as a species. Over the millennia, "humans evolved a strong appetite for sweet-tasting foods," claims the *American Journal of Clinical Nutrition.* Once upon a time, the only way we could consume carbs was through "whole, natural, seasonal, and indigenous fruits and vegetables." And when we did, we were also rewarded with mega-doses of nutrition and healthy, balanced energy.

Not anymore, thanks to the industrial age. Food manufacturers now use technology to produce highly refined carbs that are inexpensive to make and may be harmful—yet oh so appetizing. To make this test tube food, scientists engineer products to have just the right amount of sweetness to make you crave more...and more...and then stick it in everything from soft drinks to sauces. That's why the ingredients list on some of your favorite foods reads like a chemistry final. It's mad science. And we've gone mad for it. And with that manipulated food comes manipulative marketing. Foods filled with sugar are often given a "health halo"—called "all natural" or "fat free," to imply a benefit where there is none. Worst of all, unhealthy foods are targeted at children. Why else would there be cartoon characters on cereal boxes that are placed low on supermarket aisle shelving to meet kids' eyes.

As a child—and even in my early twenties—I didn't worry about any of this stuff. I certainly wasn't thinking about brain health or skin problems or inflammation or long-term effects. At that age, you think you're immortal and that you have all the time in the world to course-correct.

The truth is, the damage you're doing to your body starts years—even decades—before it strikes in any conspicuous way. If you're in your twenties and thirties, you're likely doing harm that you'll feel years from now. Lifestyle choices matter. One feature article we did at *Women's Health* really stands out in my mind. It was about the increase in "skinny diabetes" and it explained how even young, slim women are getting Type 2 diabetes, due mostly to lifestyle choices such as eating a consistently unhealthy diet and not exercising enough. Alarming stuff. The point is, you don't have to be obese to be compromising your health. And you don't have to be overweight to have a sugar problem. More important, it is never too late to take action.

My **Sugar Free 3** light bulb moment was when I realized that of all the things I'm good at mitigating and controlling, sugar is the one that has the tightest grip on me. I can bypass the pasta (when not in Italy!). I no longer eat monstrous bagels. But I'm hard-pressed to go to the movies and not mindlessly scarf down a box of candy while staring at the big screen. And after the holidays, or the end of summer, I've maxed out my sugar consumption. I can feel it.

That's why I wanted to write this book and develop this program. And when I started sharing what I was up to, every single person I told shrieked, "I need that!" Not surprising. Overeating sugar is a near-universal issue.

Again, this isn't necessarily meant to be something you strictly adhere to long term, though that wouldn't be a terrible idea. The longer you do it, the more benefits you'll reap. I just want to be honest about how I use the plan. I am by no means a "perfect" eater...there is no such thing. I eat healthfully 80 percent of the time, and the other 20 percent, I indulge. I am certainly not giving up wine for life!

The amazing thing is, now that the **Sugar Free 3** plan exists, we can return to it whenever we need a little extra guidance and support. And thanks to the ingredient education you get from this program and the healthy habits you'll be asked to institute, the positive changes will likely have staying power. You'll learn to enjoy eating mindfully and begin to recognize real hunger cues, which will help you resist cravings. (For example, you won't automatically reach for chocolate the second you finish the last bite of dinner.) You'll approach every meal a little differently and a little more thoughtfully. And yes, you can even shed excess pounds, more healthily and easily than in the past.

I'm passionate about sharing this program because I know it works, and I'm thrilled that you made the choice to give it a go! Trust me, you can do anything for three weeks.

SUGAR FREE 3 SNAPSHOT

These are the essential things to remember:

▶ *It's short! Only three weeks!*

▶ *You'll never feel hungry.*

▶ *There's no calorie counting or portion control.*

▶ *You'll eat delicious foods from the ALLOWED list like:*
  • Healthy proteins
  • Beans and legumes
  • Veggies of all kinds
  • Healthy fats
  • Whole fruit
  • Full-fat and reduced-fat dairy
  • Whole wheat and whole grain pasta, wraps and bread
  • And other NSA (no sugar added) products

▶ *Enjoy a Mindful Indulgence once a week*

▶ *You'll avoid foods from the NOT ALLOWED list:*
  • Added sugars
  • Refined carbs
  • Artificial sweeteners

▶ *Carbs are allowed!*

▶ *I developed three ways to follow the plan:*
  • Like to Cook—make our recipes or yours
  • Willing to Cook—semi-homemade using pre-prepped foods
  • Don't Cook—eat out, order in or take out

▶ *Exercise is optional.*

*Read on for all the details about how to make **Sugar Free 3** work for you.*

We're in This Together

Misery loves company. I'm kidding! But seriously, the buddy system does have benefits. Here are three steps you can take to find the support you'll need.

STEP 1

JOIN OUR COMMUNITY—STAT!

Studies have proven that people who have support and participate in "support groups" have better results than people who don't. Our test groups for **Sugar Free 3** were all part of our online community and it was amazingly helpful. Not just the results and losing 5-10-15 pounds or more in 3 weeks or sharing meal ideas, recipes and food finds but the daily support for conquering cravings and thwarting food temptation. Having thousands of people going through the process just like you, cheering you on and relating to your triumphs (and tribulations) can make a huge difference. "I work in a place that serves alcohol," said test panelist Mario C. during his first week, "and we're encouraged to try new beers. So that was interesting. But everybody knows that I'm on this challenge. So there's an expectation—and an understanding—that for a few weeks, I'll be taking a pass on the chugging. I told all my friends, and posted regularly in the **Sugar Free 3** group, where I got fist-bump emojis every time I shared a win. My co-workers also cheered me on—even if some acted like my dog just died. No sugar? You poor thing."

*Join our community. Find out more details at Openfit.com/**SF3***

STEP 2

INVITE A FRIEND

Tell your friends, spouse or co-workers about **Sugar Free 3** and see if anyone wants to do it with you. I bet you could easily round up a group—so many people consume too much sugar. There are so many reasons to do it together; you're helping them be healthier, it's more fun, you have built-in support, better focus, less distraction, less peer pressure and fewer sugar pushers (more on that in a second), you can share meal ideas, answer and solve each other's questions, eat together and support each other if you have any challenges or rough days.

STEP 3

DESIGNATE A SUGAR SPONSOR

I was walking by Dylan's Candy Bar—a brightly colored emporium of bins filled with every conceivable candy—when I felt a magnetic force trying to drag me in. I was about to cave, so I messaged my friend Allie to text me off the sugar-temptation ledge. It worked—*whew.*

My advice: to help avoid close calls like these, designate one person to be your Sugar Sponsor. Select someone in your life who's always there for you, the friend or family member who wants you to be your best self, and wants you to live your best life. Tell them you're on the **Sugar Free 3** program, and ask them to be on call for you.

Bonus points if they've successfully adhered to an eating plan in the past and know what it's like to teeter on the edge. Even better: Recruit this person to do **Sugar Free 3** with you so you have shared goals. Having a wingman or wingwoman who is living a healthy lifestyle makes all the difference. The research proves it: Overweight people tend to drop more pounds if they spend time with their healthy pals, according to a study published in the *Journal of Social Sciences.* They lose more weight the longer they hang out together. Your Sugar Sponsor is your accountability partner—and the last thing you want to do is to let him or her down. And when the going gets tough, they'll make sure *you* keep going.

Simply put, the more people who know you're on this three-week journey, the more support you'll have. It will also prevent you from having to explain yourself each time you need to place a special dinner order, suddenly start taking your coffee sans sweetener, or shockingly (in my case) refuse that glass of wine.

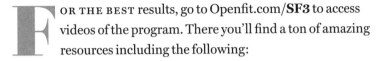

xx, Michele

Optimize With Openfit!

FOR THE BEST results, go to Openfit.com/**SF3** to access videos of the program. There you'll find a ton of amazing resources including the following:

► A series of short and informative videos led by me, teaching all the foods you can eat, how to read nutrition labels, ways to meal prep, dining out tips, plus recipes and more.

► Daily inspiration. Tune in every day for my motivational tips and pep talks to keep you going.

► Access to our community filled with people on the same journey as you to support you every step of the way! I'll be in there too!

► Extensive food lists with every edible thing you can imagine.

► A dining out guide for all your favorite cuisines.

► Hundreds of delicious **Sugar Free 3**–approved recipes.

► A customizable 21-day meal planner and tracking app to take out all of the guesswork and decision making.

► Movement and visualization videos specifically designed for this program.

► The entire Openfit video library with hundreds of workouts and Openfit Live trainer-led small group classes.

CHAPTER

1

REVEAL A WHOLE NEW YOU

How This Plan Can Help
Improve Your Life in Dramatic Ways

HOCOLATE, COOKIES, ICE CREAM, my beloved sour gummies. Just the mention of a decadent dessert or crave-worthy candy probably makes your mouth water and your pupils dilate with desire. That sense of irresistibility you feel is not your imagination (or a lack of willpower). Sugar's powers of seduction are a scientific fact—consumption of the sweet substance is known to release dopamine and endorphins, two hormones that directly increase your happiness.

But every "sugar high" has its crash. The good feelings it promotes never last—and, in fact, often end up making you feel way worse than before you indulged. That's why ditching it—even just for three weeks—can be incredibly beneficial. "When you live a sugar-free lifestyle, you'll reduce cravings for sweets, have more stable blood sugar, feel sharper and more focused and experience fewer energy and mood fluctuations," says renowned dietitian Keri Glassman, MS, RD, CDN, and founder of Nutritious Life. "There's a clear connection, especially if you target added sugars, which is exactly what this plan does."

Keri is a longtime friend and colleague, and I could think of no one better to consult with for **Sugar Free 3**. On this plan, you'll learn to easily identify which foods have added sugars and which don't. Cutting them from your diet can help you look—and, more important, feel—healthier. If you don't believe me, trust the research. Here are some of the ways you'll benefit from **Sugar Free 3**.

MORE ENERGY

I F WE ALL had food therapists, they would likely encourage us to explore the first unhealthy relationship we ever developed—with sugar. As children, we associate it with special occasions, parties, fun, rewards for good behavior, and consolation during tough times. (What did you get after a trip to the dentist? A lollipop! Oh, the irony.) Unfortunately, for most of us, that mind-set carries over into adulthood and we end up using sugar as an emotional crutch. We turn to it to fill the void after a romantic split or for self-soothing following a brutal work week. And we rely on it for a cheap, fast energy boost.

"There's a natural desire for sugar because eating it is part of an innate survival mechanism," says Keri. "When we were under stress in caveman days—say, from running away from an animal predator—we'd expend a lot of energy. To replenish that energy, we'd look for natural sugar in the form of something like berries to provide immediate fuel. The problem nowadays is that we're stressed, but we're sitting on our butts at desks or on the sofa and we don't need to hunt for fuel—it's sitting in front of us, in the form of processed, refined sugar. And when we have too much of that in our body, it gets stored as fat."

So we chow down on sugary treats to feel energized temporarily. But the reality is, in adulthood the sugar high is a fallacy—it's actually more likely to make us sleepy. Several studies show that orexin, a brain chemical that makes you feel awake, is inhibited when you eat sugar. (The after-lunch slump is real!) A June 2019 meta-analysis of 31 studies published in the journal *Neuroscience & Behavioral Reviews* found that simple carbohydrates like sugar decrease alertness and increase fatigue within an hour of consuming them.

The less alert we feel, the less physical activity we want to do—and since Americans are scarfing more sugar than ever, it's no wonder that we're the heaviest we've ever been.

That's where **Sugar Free 3** comes in. The longer you follow it, the better you'll feel. Once you finish the first three weeks, you may just want to continue this new way of eating to keep feeling amazing.

"Wait, I Have to Give Up *All* Sugar?" No!

It's nearly impossible to completely eliminate sugar from your diet. "Our brains need sugar to survive—natural sugar," says Keri. These natural sugars appear in many healthy and essential foods, such as fruits and vegetables, which are permitted on **Sugar Free 3**. The natural sugar breaks down into blood glucose—an important source of energy that your brain and body need throughout the day. "But," emphasizes Keri, "we don't need *added* sugars." That's why **Sugar Free 3** specifically targets added sugars, refined carbs, any other sugars stripped of their fiber (fruit juice, molasses, and honey, for example) and artificial sweeteners. Basically, it all comes down to this: Carbohydrates minus their fiber equals bad for your bod.

"I Lost 16 Pounds! And It's So Easy."

NAME: **JUDY G.**

AGE: **45**

HOMETOWN: **NORWALK, CALIFORNIA**

JUDY G. NEVER really had to worry about her weight—until she started having children. Three back-to-back pregnancies definitely took their toll on her body, but it wasn't something she noticed until her youngest child turned five.

"I never really thought about what I was eating, and how it was impacting my weight and overall well-being," she admits.

She relied on sugar and sugar substitutes to get through the day. Every night around 9:30 p.m., after eating dinner with her family, she looked forward to drinking a cup of coffee accompanied by a sweet treat—such as a doughnut, ice cream, or blueberry muffin. She also drank a lot of diet sodas, not because she was trying to lose weight, but because she liked the way they tasted. "I just really didn't know any better, as I was never really focused on nutrition," she confesses.

However, one day she heard about **Sugar Free 3** and was intrigued—especially because it didn't involve calorie counting or meal portioning. An added bonus? It lasted a matter of weeks. "It might actually be doable," she thought to herself—even with everything she had going on.

Almost immediately, she noticed her skin had started to improve. She learned to reduce her cravings. She also had way more energy. "I don't get so angry as fast," Judy admits. "I am just a lot happier and less moody!" She also lost 16 pounds after 2 rounds.

"It is so easy. I can eat whatever I want, when I want it, as long as there is no sugar. It's a game changer."

BETTER MOODS

THERE ARE FEW things I find more insulting than being called moody. I mean, it's like being compared to a cranky kid—for good reason. Moodiness is often the result of having consumed too much added sugar. In addition to lower energy levels, your daily sugar intake could cause mood swings—everything from rolling your eyes at your boss (not so smart) to road rage (kinda dangerous) to something way more damaging. A 2017 study published in the journal *Scientific Reports* found that high sugar consumption correlates with depression. Researchers found that people who ate a diet higher in sugar were 23 percent more likely to be depressed.

So not only will reducing sugar in your diet help with your energy—and I'll show you how a sugar-free diet can be satisfying with energizing, protein-rich foods—taking control can help make you feel less anxious and more rational. In other words, you'll feel empowered, the best mood booster there is.

REDUCED INFLAMMATION

I'M NOT TALKING about the kind you get from a bee sting or stubbed toe. The consumption of too much refined or added sugars may cause low-grade inflammation—irritation and swelling throughout the body—and over time, that can lead to a negative cycle that can have serious consequences. "Sugar causes inflammation, and inflammation is connected to most bad health conditions," says Keri. "It's a huge problem and the reason sugar is probably the worst thing in our diets."

The impact is quantifiable: A study in the *American Journal of Clinical Nutrition* found that when healthy young men consumed just one sugar-sweetened beverage containing 40 grams of sugar (about the same as a 12-ounce soda) per day for three weeks, their bodies experienced an increase in their C-reactive protein—a known inflammation marker.

To understand why, I need to relay a short biology lesson—stick with me. Once you swallow a bite of sugary food, it lands in your stomach and is exposed to your digestive juices and moves more quickly from your stomach to your small intestine than other types of food. There, it's broken down with digestive enzymes and turned into monosaccharide, a single-molecule form of sugar. These single molecules are secreted through the small intestine and absorbed into your bloodstream as glucose.

In small doses, this is perfectly acceptable, but when your blood sugar goes too high and your insulin spikes (which happens with fast-absorbing sugars and refined carbohydrates), your immune system responds by creating pro-inflammatory proteins called cytokines to help combat the situation. The low-grade inflammation your body experiences when you overconsume added sugars can put it under stress and lead to poor health. By eliminating added sugars from your diet, your gut can better perform its essential function as gatekeeper. This helps reduce the tax on your body. You'll chill out—and your body gets a break too.

Pushing the Sugar Limits

According to the American Heart Association (AHA), the maximum amount of added sugars you should eat in a day are:

- **MEN:**
  150 calories per day
  (37.5 grams or 9 teaspoons)

- **WOMEN:**
  100 calories per day
  (25 grams or 6 teaspoons)

Just one 12-ounce can of regular soda contains eight teaspoons of sugar, or 130 calories and zero nutrition, says the AHA. Yup, just one can of soda can put women over the limit.

Said another way, less than 10 percent of your daily calorie intake should come from added sugars, according to government regulations. And yet a brand new study from Tufts say 42 percent of our daily calories come from low-quality carbohydrates like refined grains and added sugars.

HEALTHIER-LOOKING SKIN

WORRIED ABOUT WRINKLES? Obsessed with your complexion? I am. In fact, I'm on a constant quest for better skin and I practically live to try new products, which I constantly got to do as a magazine editor. I'm a bit of a product junkie. (The beauty closet in my office was my happy place.) But excessive sugar can derail efforts to have compliment-worthy skin.

"There are multiple biological reasons to explain the connection, but one that stands out is the effects that refined carbs have on spiking blood sugar, which in turn can also increase hormones that stimulate oil production," explains Whitney Bowe, MD, one of the most in-demand dermatologists in the country and author of the bestselling book *Dirty Looks: The Secret to Beautiful Skin*. I am lucky enough to have her as my personal dermatologist and, now, friend. I asked her about how sugar can impact skin health. "These hormones can even change the composition of your skin's oil," says Dr. Bowe, "making it more prone to issues."

Dr. Bowe says sugar causes issues that are more than skin deep, triggering "multiple changes in our body, from our cellular membranes and our arteries to our hormones, immune systems, gut microbiome—the microbes in our intestines that affect our biology all the way out to our skin." Dr. Bowe goes on to say, "One big reason to avoid too much sugar is that it has a direct hit on skin thanks to glycation."

This science fascinates me: Glycation is when sugar molecules bond to protein or fat molecules to create something called "glycation end products," or AGEs. (Fitting, don't you think?) These AGEs inhibit elasticity in all kinds of bodily tissues, including your skin. In other words, they can cause premature wrinkles. The scientists call this "sugar sag." Eek!

One factor in creating AGEs is having too much glucose and fructose in your diet. This glycation doesn't just appear as crow's feet or frown lines. Once consumed, excessive sugar wreaks havoc on your entire body, and both glucose and fructose (fruit sugar, another monosaccharide) are absorbed into all of your body tissues. Glycation creates these AGEs in the skin all over, and their effects are only exacerbated by the sun's UV rays. Your skin becomes less elastic and appears to age more rapidly.

"To see AGEs in action, simply look at someone who is prematurely aging—someone with a lot of wrinkles, sagginess, discolored skin, and a loss of radiance for their age," says Dr. Bowe. "What you're seeing is the physical effect of proteins latching on to renegade sugars. Scientists can document a parallel in animal research between how much sugar they consume and how fast their skin ages. More sugar equates with 'older looking' skin that has lost its elasticity and suppleness prematurely."

Reducing your consumption of added sugars, as you will on **Sugar**

By the Numbers

In an initial test group, 25 **Sugar Free 3** users went through the program and told us about the benefits they experienced. Here are their results:*

| 0% | 25% | 50% | 75% | 100% |

LESS BLOATING: 48%

MORE ENERGY: 80%

LOST WEIGHT: 100%

LOST OVER 5 LBS: 52%

LOST OVER 10 LBS: 24%

REDUCED CRAVINGS: 88%

MORE SELF-CONTROL: 96%

NOTICEABLE SKIN IMPROVEMENTS: 56%

BETTER SLEEP: 20%

EXCITED TO KEEP IT GOING: 100%

*The test group included independent users and
Openfit, LLC employees completing the entire **Sugar Free 3** program.

Free 3, can help improve your skin's tone, elasticity and overall appearance. You'll walk into every room feeling confident, putting your best face (and neck, and arms, and legs) forward. "My skin is so clear," reported Trinity A., who tested the program. "For me, there's nothing more exciting that walking by a mirror and feeling good. When you feel good, you look good, and when you look good, you feel good."

SHARPER FOCUS

OUR BRAINS have a love/hate relationship with sugar, says another pal of mine, Max Lugavere, author of the *New York Times* bestselling book *Genius Foods* and host of the health podcast *The Genius Life*. "The brain loves sugar—it needs it to run smoothly, and it's pleasurable," he says, adding, "but it's exponentially more pleasurable when it's added to packaged, processed foods, which we now eat with abandon. And when we overconsume these types of foods, the brain might not work as well."

When Max and I first met, we bonded over the fact that both of our moms have struggled with cognitive issues—and we are both committed to doing what we can to thwart suffering that same fate and to help others do the same. (You can find our info-packed conversation on the Openfit app.) There's plenty of research out there backing up the deteriorative impact sugar can have, including one study in the *Journal of Alzheimer's Disease* that associated mild cognitive impairment with elderly people who ate a diet high in carbs and low in protein and fat. Another study in *Clinical Interventions in Aging* surveyed more than 1,200 adults over the age of 60 and found an association between "excessive sugar consumption" and poor cognitive function.

But sugar issues don't just kick in with old age. A study in the *British Journal of Nutrition* of more than 7,000 people between the ages of

45 and 70 also linked higher sugar intake with a decline in cognitive function. The study didn't determine whether excessive sugar consumption caused a lack of brain power or a lack of brain power caused excessive sugar consumption. Either way, less sharp people tended to eat too much sugar.

Luckily, I know I'm writing to a smart crowd here.

If you're sick of feeling foggy, or you feel like you're losing focus during the day, I can report that those who did **Sugar Free 3** swear it helped clear their heads.

IMPROVED DIGESTION

DURING MY YEARS as a wellness editor, I have reported on countless new discoveries. One stands apart from the rest in terms of the attention paid and game-changing light that exploring it has shed on health and well-being. I'm talking about the gut microbiome. In the last few years, no fewer than 25 books have been written about gut health. You don't need to read any of them right now because I am going to CliffsNotes it for you here.

Your gut microbiome contains trillions of bacteria, with hundreds of different species fighting for dominance. We know the "good" ones play a vital role in digestion, help modulate your immune system, and help fight off pathogens—but that's just the start. Research is emerging every day suggesting that your gut plays an even bigger role in keeping the rest of your body and your mind in peak condition.

Fortunately, science is catching up quickly on how to best feed these little wonder bugs. We know that certain kinds of fibers called prebiotics help, as do probiotics (live microorganisms found in certain supplements and foods). What's not on the menu for a healthy gut microbiome? You guessed it—sugar!

Proof of this digestion-blocking dilemma is contained in a recent report in the *Proceedings of the National Academy of Sciences,* which showed that heavy doses of fructose and glucose (which combine to make sucrose, aka "table sugar") can block the growth of *Bacteroides thetaiotamicron,* which is a bacterium often found in the guts of people who maintain a balanced diet and a healthy weight. Simply put: It helps you digest dietary fiber properly.

So when you steer clear of excessive sugar in your diet, your gut can retain its natural function. With a full staff and a healthy environment, your gut flora can get to work keeping your digestive system—just to name one thing—running smoothly.

HOTTER SEX

No NEED TO blush. I was the Editor-in-Chief of *Cosmopolitan* so I'm somewhat of an authority on this endlessly fascinating subject. Even if you haven't read *Cosmo,* no doubt you've seen some of the attention-grabbing sex coverlines. Every cover we did mentioned sex, because most people want more of it—or at least more satisfaction from it.

One thing my readers were surprised to learn is that what happens between the sheets is linked to what goes down in their kitchens (and I'm not talking about some impromptu countertop romp). High consumption of sugar negatively affects your energy levels, and we all know how a lack of energy can impact your desire to get busy. Lethargy and lack of get-up-and-go is a major reason why sex lives fizzle out, especially for long-term couples.

And if you're a guy, consuming excess sugar may have an even more dampening effect on your mojo. According to a 2018 study published in the journal *Reproductive Biology and Endocrinology,* men who consumed sugar-sweetened beverages had a lower testosterone level than those who abstained from those drinks.

Want to know my number one tip for more energy and better performance? Kick the sugar out of bed!

Sugar-Free Foods for Better Sex

Chocolate and champagne might have a rep for being aphrodisiacs, but their sugar content is more likely to turn you off than on. Here are some foods that will heat up your next date night.

CHILI PEPPERS

Add some serrano peppers to a stir fry, jalapeños to guacamole, or cayenne pepper to your eggs. Each pepper contains a significant amount of capsaicin (the compound that makes hot sauce hot), which releases chemicals that increase heart rate, mirror signs of arousal, and release feel-good endorphins.

AVOCADOS

Your anxiety about getting between the sheets could be elevating levels of stress—which plummet libido. And a lack of B-vitamins—nutrients that keep nerves and brain cells healthy—could also be exaggerating your stress even further, says a *Nutrition Journal* study. The solution? Feast on some guac to take advantage of the fact that avocados are a good source of B vitamins.

GINGER

If you like your food like you like your lovers—sweet and spicy—you're in luck. According to a study in the *International Journal of Cardiology*, consuming a mere teaspoon of ginger a few times a week is all you need to reap the heart-healthy benefits.

SOUNDER SLEEP

WHEN I WAS a little girl, all I wanted to do was stay up late and watch TV like the big kids and adults. When I was in college, I'd pull all-nighters (and sometimes even study during them). And during my twenties and thirties, Manhattan—the city that never sleeps—lived up to its tagline, causing me to spend way too many evenings out until the wee hours thanks to my FOMO (Fear of Missing Out). And that was before the term FOMO even existed!

Now I realize that what I was missing out on was more important than any DJ spinning at a club—quality sleep. Sleep is a key player in the brain's regulation of appetite and energy levels. That's why getting seven to nine hours is critically important. It's another thing health journalist Max Lugavere has impressed upon me. "Just a 30-minute deficit can disrupt your metabolism," says Max, leading to a slower burn rate of calories, not to mention more cravings. (It can lead to a whole host of health issues, too.)

That's why I was thrilled to hear that people who tried **Sugar Free 3** reported falling asleep more easily on the plan. They even reported getting better sleep. And it is one of the benefits I personally noticed early on when I started eating sugar free. It makes sense. Without added sugars sparking a short-term "energy" boost before bedtime, we're able to drift off naturally, leading to steadier energy levels when it matters most: during the day!

STRONGER AWARENESS

FEELING IN CONTROL of your own destiny is one of the most liberating states there is. A meaningful way to get there is to take the reins of your diet. Just like in romantic partnerships or an exercise regimen, it's easy to sink into a rut with our eating patterns and relationship to food. Over the next few weeks you will become much more aware and mindful of the foods you eat. And you may realize that you have been mindlessly eating when tired, happy, sad, stressed, or simply off your routine. So many of us have defaulted to unhealthy habits that aren't serving us or even particularly enjoyable. In **Sugar Free 3**, you will also learn to replace do-nothing foods with satisfying, nutritious alternatives. I know that within days you will feel changes and start seeing results because you took control.

AND EASIER WEIGHT LOSS, TOO!

I T'S THE RARE person who doesn't want to drop a few pounds. And giving up added sugars can help—big time. I dropped six or so pounds—enough to peel off the excess I'd put on from a gluttonous vacation to Italy, where gelato became a staple of my diet. The beauty of **Sugar Free 3** is that you don't have to portion out your food, count calories, or (most awesome of all) ever be hungry. And it's highly likely you'll lose weight.

Max notes one of the reasons why losing a little may seem more effortless on **SF3**: "Giving up sugar for three weeks can help you start to 'reset' your palette so that you are less likely to even crave sweet foods," says Max. "You'll also be consuming fewer empty calories since sugar has no nutritional value. This should help you lose weight and also increase your nutritional status since you'll be making up for the sugar you aren't eating with real, whole foods."

"For anyone struggling with weight issues, lack of willpower, or even just fatigue and low energy, cutting out sources of added sugar can be a great way of boosting health and getting on the road to wellness," adds Max. When you start eating nutritious, satisfying meals like the ones

I recommend on this program, you'll feel more satisfied. Think about how many calories you can save just by cutting out two sodas a day, that coffee with cream and sugar, and your afternoon chocolate fix. (Let's be honest, can anyone really stop at just one square?) That could amount to a pound a week! Plus, when you eat sugar, you tend to crave sugary foods. When you start cutting back, you'll notice that you miss sugary treats less and less.

It's pretty simple. Follow the plan: Eat less sugar. Fill up on satisfying foods with healthy fats, nutrients, protein, and fiber your body needs. And without realizing it, you'll eat fewer calories, which can help you drop weight and shrink your waistline. Read on to discover how well it worked for our test group.

And, if weight-loss is your top goal, there are some bonus insights I want to share to help you reach your ultimate goal. You'll find those in Chapter 6, dedicated to accelerating weight loss—the healthy way.

CHAPTER

2

END YOUR DEPENDENCE ON SUGAR

And Its Evil Twins:
Refined Carbs and Artificial Sweeteners!

S A MAGAZINE EDITOR, I worked on my fair share of articles about unhealthy relationships—and thanks to that, I'm able to spot the perpetrators a lot more easily now. But there's one type that's sneakier than the rest: The frenemy. And that's exactly what sugar is.

Sure, it acts like your most supportive BFF—there for you at all hours, especially the late ones when you think you need it most. But when you stop to really think about it, sugar takes way more than it gives. It expects—no, demands!—an immediate response to every call for attention. And hanging with it too much messes with your skin, mood, and weight. It's time to end your attachment to this selfish sidekick.

As with any bad relationship, you might be asking yourself: "How did I let this happen?" Well, I'm here to tell you that it's not your fault. In this chapter, you'll learn the difference between sugar, refined carbs, and artificial sweeteners, how they hurt us, and the multitude of factors—from societal pressures to personal genetics to food manufacturers—that got you here. And then I'll tell you how to break free. Let me first explain the difference:

- ◆ **Added Sugars** / add·ed sug·ars / *n*. Sugars added to foods when they are prepared or processed—as opposed to the naturally occurring sugar in, say, an apple or a glass of milk.

- ◆ **Refined Carbs** / re·fined carbs / *n*. Processed foods that have been stripped of nutrients. For example, to make white bread, manufacturers remove the outer coating of a wheat kernel (known as the bran) and the germ—the good stuff. Only the inner endosperm is then ground into flour.

- ◆ **Artificial Sweeteners** / ar·ti·fi·cial sweet·en·ers / *n*. Chemicals added to foods to make them taste sweeter, with little to no caloric (or nutritional) value. They can be hundreds of times sweeter than sugar.

SUGAR AND OBESITY

EXCESSIVE SUGAR consumption is linked to significant and damaging health effects.

Obesity

Researchers warn that too much sugar leads to obesity. In 2016, the CDC concluded that 93.3 million American adults, or 39.8 percent, were considered obese.

"Sugar is just empty calories," says Max Lugavere. Because of that, it makes you more likely to want to eat other unhealthy foods to attempt to satisfy your hunger. Additionally, "sugar is often found in the worst place—where you'll also find unhealthy oils and chemicals," adds Keri Glassman.

And as previously noted, you experience chemical and emotional responses to sugar consumption that can make you overeat and gain weight. A study published in *Frontiers of Psychiatry* asked 19 people to consume one 10-ounce sugary drink each. After consuming, they were shown photos of high-calorie, processed, sugary foods, like pizza and ice cream. They showed heightened responses to these photos and a reduced level of GLP-1, a hormone responsible for appetite suppression, when compared with the placebo group.

Another study conducted by the American Diabetes Association found that when adults and children lowered their intake of sugary drinks, they lost weight.

Worse yet, obesity is linked to other alarming health conditions that are caused by carrying too much weight, including:

◆ *Type 2 diabetes* ◆ *Certain types of cancer*

◆ *High blood pressure* ◆ *Fatty liver disease*

◆ *Stroke* ◆ *Kidney disease*

◆ *Heart disease* ◆ *Osteoarthritis*

What you think causes a heart attack—red meat or faulty genetics, right?—may be out of date. According to the National Institute of Diabetes and Digestive and Kidney Diseases, losing just 5 to 10 percent of your overall body weight can lower your chances of developing heart disease. A study published in *JAMA Internal Medicine* found that a high-sugar diet was linked to increased risk of dying from heart disease. Participants who consumed 17 percent to 21 percent of their daily calories from added sugar were studied over the course of 15 years. They were found to have a 38 percent higher risk of dying from cardiovascular disease than participants who only consumed 8 percent of their daily calories from added sugars.

HOW WE GOT HERE

DON'T WORRY, I'M not going to give you yawn-inducing lessons on the Harrowing History of Horrible Foods. But the following bullet points are worth breezing through.

- Sugar was once considered a luxury item in Europe for kings, queens, and the elite. Christopher Columbus brought sugar cane to the Dominican Republic in 1492—the first time it landed on this side of the world.

- It quickly "went viral" in the Caribbean and South America, and the early settlers soon realized they couldn't keep up with demand. They needed workers to plant fields and harvest the crops.

- Here's where things get ugly. This "white gold" quickly became the fuel that drove the slave trade. Plantations covered America, the Caribbean, and most of South America.

- By the 1700s, sugar was a huge economic boom in America—and continued to be one of the driving forces of slavery, with production exploding in the South. The Revolutionary War resulted in America's independence, and you likely know the highlights of the last 250 or so years. All along, we produced more and more sugar.

- In the 1940s, we also produced more refined carbs. Companies used new machinery—some inspired by World War II—to make foods faster and cheaper.

- In 1957, high fructose corn syrup (HFCS) was invented—in part to find a use for all the corn American farmers were growing. From 1975 to 1985, it was rapidly added to a wide spectrum of processed foods, largely to support the corn industry. "Corn" sounded healthier than sugar. Decades later, we learned that HFCS, just like sugar, was a prime culprit in the obesity epidemic.

◆ Artificial sweeteners also boomed in the 1950s, thanks to the diet soda craze. They also sounded "healthier" than sugar.

◆ The sweet stuff is now harvested with machines, but its shady history lives on in every culture it touched. All these years later, Brazil is currently the number one sugar cane producing country. The U.S. is tenth—but we consume more sugar than any country in the world.

In whatever form, food makers were ready for the sugar boom and more than happy to cash in. Sugar, the "nutrient," was originally slipped into packaged food by manufacturers to make it more appealing and better tasting, according to a study published in *Frontiers in Psychiatry*. Since packaged foods are usually the cheapest to produce and the cheapest to buy, their popularity exploded. By the nineteenth century, foods were marketed by their flavor combinations, colors, brand names, and convenient packaging. What used to be important about food—its nutritional value, ingredients, and origin—were no longer discussed or promoted.

Eating sugar became a new way of life. And you likely don't remember a time when it wasn't. Most people ate sugar every day and fed it to their families. Remember how I recounted that the pantry and fridge of my childhood home was jam-packed with sugary cereals and chocolaty drinks? We were not alone! No one preached about the dangers, but these foods—coupled with our increasingly sedentary lifestyles—are what led us to become the unhealthy Americans we are today.

Most of these sugars are added sugars—the sugar carbs added

to foods during production. Less than 10 percent of your daily calorie intake should come from added sugars, according to government regulations. And yet a brand new study from Tufts University say 42 percent of our daily calories come from low-quality carbohydrates like refined grains and added sugars.

TOO GOOD NOT TO EAT

BEYOND ITS LOW cost, sugar is enticing for other reasons: "It creates a pleasing mouth-feel and tastes impossibly delicious when combined with other ingredients, like fat and salt," says health journalist Max Lugavere. "Sugar is complicit in the hyperpalatable nature of packaged foods, which are easy to overconsume—they're so tasty and convenient—and yet they are not satiating at all."

It's true, food manufacturers (or Big Food, as the collective is referred to) spend countless dollars on research and development to create foods that taste so good and feel so right in your mouth that you become a reliable repeat customer.

But we also crave sugar because it's a quick fix of sweetness in a sometimes bitter world, at least according to advertisers who bombard us with marketing messages that hammer away at how much we deserve to eat something sweet. And that's not all. Dopamine is a neurotransmitter within your body's "reward center." When you do something your body gets a charge from, dopamine is the chemical that's released in your brain that makes you feel good—and that makes you want to keep doing it. When dopamine is released while you're eating a piece of chocolate, it's responsible for that persuasive voice inside your head telling you to start breaking off the next bite.

"A lot of us have developed a sugar dependence—feeling sugar highs and lows," says registered dietitian Keri Glassman, who explains: "The

"I'm Absolutely in Love With This Feeling!"

NAME: MARIO C.

AGE: 24

HOMETOWN: EL SEGUNDO, CALIFORNIA

"ABS ARE MADE in the kitchen," goes the popular slogan. Especially if that kitchen is sugar-free. In 21 days, Mario C., a bartender/DJ, lost 7.6 lbs while doing **Sugar Free 3**, and got a six-pack in the process. Combining the meal plan with cardio and weight-training four days a week, he was able to shed fat where he wanted to lose it most. "I feel so different than I did three weeks ago," he told me at the end of the program. "I have more muscle definition all over my body, and noticed less puffiness in my face. And I have more energy."

His physical transformation was impressive. But I was also thrilled by the power of his new outlook. "I have so much more mental strength," Mario said. "I definitely don't have the same desire for processed junk food as before. Fresh fruit tastes so much better than a candy bar now. The most pivotal thing I noticed was my overall energy has increased. I really feel super all the time and I'm absolutely in love with this feeling. I feel stronger and sharper and therefore more confident."

Mario says he'll "absolutely" continue the program past the 21 days. "I loved the support and guidance of the group," he added, referring to the type of community you'll find at openfit.com/**SF3**. "It felt like a little fit family, and it's definitely easier and more exciting to be health-conscious when there are other people in your corner. I am 100 percent ready to keep it going."

more we have, the more we want. And the more we have, the harder it is to get that same buzz. You want that hit of dopamine. You want to feel good. But this dependence can disrupt sleep, leading to fatigue and increased consumption of other calories, which causes a whole host of health issues."

And yet we keep consuming it. Logically, you may know that sugar

Just a Spoonful of Sugar? More Like 10.

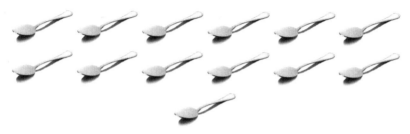

16 ounces of Coca-Cola contains 52g added sugar (13 tsp)

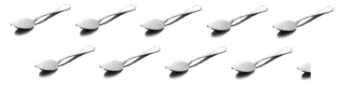

1 can Red Bull has 37g sugar (9.25 tsp)

2 tablespoons (1 serving) Wish-Bone Italian Dressing contains 4g added sugar (1 tsp)

Thomas' Plain Bagel contains 5g added sugar (1¼ tsp)

is bad and can lead to adverse effects, but your reward center drives you to just keep eating. So why do we blatantly ignore the health experts—or even our own common sense? The scary truth is, many of us don't even know when we're eating added sugars.

The U.S. Food and Drug Administration (FDA) calculated that

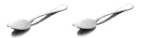

⅔ cup Kellogg's All-Bran Cereal contains 8g added sugar (2 tsp)

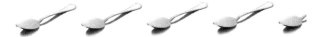

4 tablespoons (2 servings) Nestle Toll House Chocolate Chip Cookie Dough contains 18g added sugar (4½ tsp)

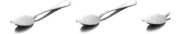

1 serving (½ pizza) California Pizza Kitchen Gluten Free Barbecue Recipe Chicken Crispy Thin Crust Pizza contains 10g added sugar (2½ tsp)

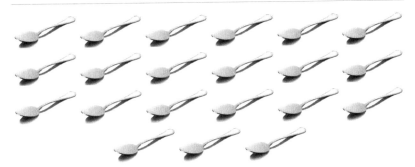

One pint of Ben and Jerry's Peanut Butter Fudge Core contains 84g added sugar (21 tsp)

All brand names and trademarks are the property of their respective owners. Information obtained from product websites as of November 2019.

there are over 60 different names used for "sugar" on food labels—
with covert monikers such as dextrose, barley malt and sucrose (for an
extensive list, see page 42).

It gets worse. Most shoppers assume they only need to look out
for added sugars in sweet foods, such as cookies and cakes. However,
added sugar, refined carbs, and artificial sweeteners are also present in
many major brands of:

- *Pasta sauce*
- *Bread*
- *Bagels*
- *Hamburger and
  hot dog buns*
- *Protein or granola bars*
- *Breakfast cereals*
- *Crackers*
- *Yogurt*
- *Canned fruits and vegetables*
- *Ketchup, barbecue sauce, etc.*
- *Dried fruits*
- *Salad dressings*

Added sugar is the original "phantom menace." Says Keri: "If you take
a look at what's in your pantry, you'll see the crackers, dressing, and
marinara sauce likely have sugar. You may have an increased desire for
sugar because you're consuming more of it than you even realize."

Of course manufacturers don't warn us of this, and they also mis-
lead us about the true nature of weight gain. "We are told that obesity
is the result of moral failure or lack of willpower," says Max. "But few of
us have adequate willpower in the face of these modern creations, and
sugar clearly plays a role."

Bottom line: Resistance may be difficult, but it's achievable when
you're armed with the right tools. You'll easily eliminate added sugars on **Sugar Free 3**, stopping this cycle of dependence. It's time to
rewrite history.

BEWARE THE HEALTH HALO

ON'T FEEL FOOLISH for getting tricked into thinking "health" foods like yogurt and granola are good for you. The food labels misled you, alluding to a food having redemptive benefits, even though they're packed with way too much sugar.

These "health halo" labels are tactics designed to get you to buy junk food without feeling bad about it. The Food and Drug Administration is constantly looking for ways to regulate the claims food manufacturers make on their packaging, but it's a little like trying to herd cats. You might see labels on food packages that say "Natural," "Light," "Diet," "Healthy," or even "Sugar Free." These claims may mean something positive, but they also distract from the negative aspects of whatever you're about to eat.

For example, one of the most common "health" food package labels you'll see is "Low-Fat" or "Fat-Free." While this may be true, it's important to keep in mind that the absence or reduction of fat usually means the presence of way too much added sugar. Manufacturers know they must make low-fat foods palatable in some way, so they add tons of unhealthy sugar to make you enjoy the product (and want more of it). What's worse is many products claim to be "sugar free" and have replaced the sugar with artificial sweetener. It's beyond lame.

Some of the most common health halo food terms are:

"Natural"

At this writing, the FDA hadn't formally defined the term "natural," but many consider it as food without artificial flavors, added colors, or synthetic ingredients. That's great, but it's also incredibly easy to sidestep. As a consumer you might think a "natural" food sounds healthy and free of processed ingredients, so you're making a great decision. In actuality, it can still contain added sugars and unhealthy ingredients.

"Organic"

With an "organic" label, the devil is in the details. A food that claims to be "100% organic" is made with all organic ingredients or foods that weren't grown or made using bioengineered genes (GMOs), synthetic pesticides, or sewage sludge–based or petroleum-based fertilizers. However, if a label simply says "Organic," it means the food is only made with 95 percent organic ingredients. If the food is labeled as "Made with Organic Ingredients," it's 70 percent organic and 30 percent of the ingredients are defined by other regulations, but aren't necessarily organic. Organic food can reduce or eliminate the chemicals you're ingesting. But these foods can still contain added and refined sugars, which doesn't always make them the healthiest choices.

I could make you an organic chocolate cake with organic sugar, organic refined flour, organic butter, organic chocolate, and organic eggs. I could even write the word "organic" on top of it in organic frosting. Would that make my cake good for you? Absolutely not.

"Gluten Free"

Gluten is a protein that occurs naturally in grains, such as wheat, rye, and barley. The FDA defines a "gluten-free" product as one that limits the presence of gluten to less than 20 parts per million (ppm). This label is helpful for celiac disease sufferers or other consumers who need to avoid ingesting gluten. However, even foods that don't naturally contain gluten can use this to trick consumers into thinking they have health benefits. Also, many people mistakenly believe that gluten-free automatically equals healthy. This allows added sugars or other unhealthy ingredients to slip by in these products unbeknownst to consumers.

"Wheat" or "Multigrain"

This is one of the biggest health halos of them all. Unless a product is labeled "whole wheat" or " whole grain," it can still be refined flour, making it as bad as simple sugar. When shopping for breads and grain products, always check the Nutrition Facts label, and aim to choose whole wheat or whole grain varieties with no added sugars, and as few ingredients as possible.

"Enriched"

"Enriched" foods sound like they have vitamins or minerals added. That's not wrong, exactly. What the labels won't tell you is that those vitamins and minerals were likely stripped away during processing and then added back in. (I remember the "enriched" white bread of my childhood; turns out the nutrients were lost due to bleaching the flour, and then tossed back in.) Furthermore, while healthy foods can be enriched, enriched foods aren't necessarily healthy.

"High Energy"

And wait—sugar itself has been crowned with the health halo of being an "energy food." This isn't a completely erroneous marketing ploy. As stated earlier, your body needs sugar (a.k.a. glucose) to provide you with energy. When you consume sugar, it's digested and enters the bloodstream, where it's delivered to your body's cells. It provides your cells with energy and helps your body to function. If it's not needed, your body stores it. However, food manufacturers are known to abuse that catchphrase. And they haven't been very quick to warn consumers of the adverse effects of eating too much added sugar, which nearly everyone does.

Energy drinks, sports drinks, and fruit-flavored waters are some of the emptiest braggarts about the energy and nutritional benefits of sugar. Think about how many times you see famous athletes marketing sugar-filled sports drinks. The manufacturer wants the consumer to attribute to these sugary drinks muscle building, performance, and endurance.

Don't get me wrong. There are times when these drinks can be beneficial. If you're quarterbacking an NCAA game or competing in an Ironman, then sure, you're going to need all the sugar and electrolytes you can get. But couch surfers and weekend gym warriors shouldn't fool themselves. To your body, it's essentially getting pretty colored sugar water.

Meanwhile, you don't see commercials about how energizing a few glasses of water and a serving or two of fruit—rich in natural sugar, satiating fiber, and health-promoting phytochemicals—can be.

In other words, the processed food industry perverts these claims into buzzwords to get your attention and raise their prices.

A BETTER FUTURE: LABELS THAT DON'T LIE

FINALLY, SOME encouraging news: the FDA is shining a spotlight on fibbers and forcing the use of the term "added sugars."

On May 27, 2016, new rules were published that required food manufacturers to change the way they label their foods. Recent findings on the link between diet and chronic conditions, including obesity and heart disease, pushed the FDA to implement these changes.

One of the most notable changes on the new label is the addition of "added sugars" under the Nutrition Facts. The FDA defines "added sugars" as sugars "that are either added during the processing of foods, or are packaged as such, and include sugars (free, mono- and disaccharides), sugars from syrups and honey, and sugars from concentrated fruit

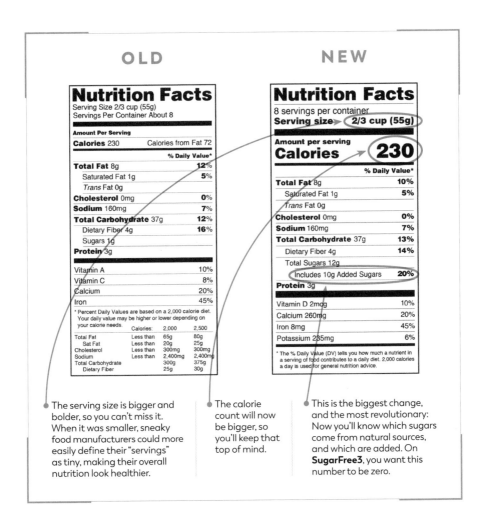

OLD

Nutrition Facts
Serving Size 2/3 cup (55g)
Servings Per Container About 8

Amount Per Serving
Calories 230 — Calories from Fat 72

% Daily Value*
Total Fat 8g — 12%
Saturated Fat 1g — 5%
Trans Fat 0g
Cholesterol 0mg — 0%
Sodium 160mg — 7%
Total Carbohydrate 37g — 12%
Dietary Fiber 4g — 16%
Sugars 1g
Protein 3g

Vitamin A — 10%
Vitamin C — 8%
Calcium — 20%
Iron — 45%

* Percent Daily Values are based on a 2,000 calorie diet. Your daily value may be higher or lower depending on your calorie needs.

	Calories:	2,000	2,500
Total Fat	Less than	65g	80g
Sat Fat	Less than	20g	25g
Cholesterol	Less than	300mg	300mg
Sodium	Less than	2,400mg	2,400mg
Total Carbohydrate		300g	375g
Dietary Fiber		25g	30g

NEW

Nutrition Facts
8 servings per container
Serving size 2/3 cup (55g)

Amount per serving
Calories **230**

% Daily Value*
Total Fat 8g — 10%
Saturated Fat 1g — 5%
Trans Fat 0g
Cholesterol 0mg — 0%
Sodium 160mg — 7%
Total Carbohydrate 37g — 13%
Dietary Fiber 4g — 14%
Total Sugars 12g
Includes 10g Added Sugars — 20%
Protein 3g

Vitamin D 2mcg — 10%
Calcium 260mg — 20%
Iron 8mg — 45%
Potassium 235mg — 6%

* The % Daily Value (DV) tells you how much a nutrient in a serving of food contributes to a daily diet. 2,000 calories a day is used for general nutrition advice.

The serving size is bigger and bolder, so you can't miss it. When it was smaller, sneaky food manufacturers could more easily define their "servings" as tiny, making their overall nutrition look healthier.

The calorie count will now be bigger, so you'll keep that top of mind.

This is the biggest change, and the most revolutionary: Now you'll know which sugars come from natural sources, and which are added. On **SugarFree3**, you want this number to be zero.

or vegetable juices that are in excess of what would be expected from the same volume of 100 percent fruit or vegetable juice of the same type."

The new label will provide the number of grams of added sugars in the product, displayed under the "Carbohydrates" heading. You can also see a percentage of the daily value for sugar, taking added sugars into account.

The FDA states it made this change because there's now enough solid published research concluding that when added sugars are consumed excessively, the diet is imbalanced. The agency worries that with too many added sugars in the diet, there isn't enough caloric intake left for other nutritious food. This can lead to a diet without enough dietary fiber, vitamins, and minerals.

The goal of the new information provided on these labels is to ensure consumers can make accurately informed choices when comparing foods. Many manufacturers have already switched to the updated label. Critical note: According to the FDA, food manufacturers with $10 million or more in annual food sales must make this nutrition label change by January 1, 2020. However, manufacturers with less than $10 million in annual food sales aren't required to change their product labels until January 1, 2021.

This new nutrition label rollout didn't come without a little controversy. Of course, the sugar industry attempted to fight back against the FDA to stop the regulation on the new label. The Sugar Association argued again that the science was wrong and misleading and that sugar just wasn't as dangerous as everyone was making it out to be.

The Sugar Association combated the FDA on the new label because it claimed that the sugar that naturally occurs in foods is the same processed byproduct food manufacturers add to products. While this is true, the association failed to mention how added sugars can dilute the nutritional value of food and provide empty calories in the American diet.

Why put up such a big fight? Likely because the sugar industry knew that if consumers had access to information on the exact amount of added sugars in their food, they'd make different and healthier choices. In turn, food manufacturers would begin to use less and less sugar in their products, taking a toll on the sugar industry's profit.

Fat Was the Fall Guy

Y NOW, YOU might be wondering how sugar was able to hide in plain sight for so many decades. The answer is, the food industry pointed the finger at another culprit: fat. Yes, they fat-shamed fat!

It all started in the 1960s, in the belly of the beast—the sugar industry. An article published in *JAMA Internal Medicine* analyzed internal sugar industry documents and concluded that the sugar industry funded research with the goal of highlighting the dangers of fat and downplaying the risks of a high-sugar diet.

The documents confirmed that an industry group called the Sugar Research Foundation had the goal of refuting current research findings that concluded there was a correlation between sugar and heart disease. To do so, the group sponsored Harvard scientists to examine and combat tons of sugar studies that proved the dangerous effects of eating too much added sugar. The scientists also provided their own report concluding that eating too much fat was unhealthy and claiming that cutting out this evil nutrient reduces the risk of coronary artery disease.

The sugar industry handpicked the studies to publish and market to the public. Can you guess which ones they picked? Studies that put sugar in a good light and made fat the enemy were marketed aggressively. It became ingrained in our brains that to be healthy, we only needed to focus on low-fat or fat-free foods. This sparked the renaissance of high-sugar and low-fat foods, which only fed into our already present overconsumption of added sugars .

What I hope to you'll learn from this program is how to identify sugar that may be hiding in your food and be an educated shopper and consumer. After three weeks you're going to approach your dining choices with a whole new perspective, from reading labels on purchases and the foods in your pantry, to ordering in, dining out, and even your own cooking.

WHAT HAVE WE LEARNED?

EXCESSIVE CONSUMPTION OF added sugars is linked to a host of negative health issues. Not only that, consuming too many foods with added sugars is simply a waste of your daily caloric intake. A consistently imbalanced diet that deprives you of essential nutrients and fiber can also be the cause of weight gain and just feeling unwell.

By eating too many sugars, you're detracting from your ability to live well. But here's the good news: It's never too late. Ditching excess added sugars from your diet now can get you on the right path to better health and wellness.

READY, SET— GO!

Here's How You'll Do **Sugar Free 3**

THIS PLAN is built on a few simple principles that anyone can follow. Once mastered, they will become second nature—forever, if you want. You'll eat foods from an Allowed list and avoid foods from a Not Allowed list. There are other guideposts, but that is the essence of the plan: Stick to the lists and **Sugar Free 3** will work for you!

I've put together this chapter to help you get started. It does require some pre-planning and ingredient education, but I'll be here for you every step of the way.

READY

PICK YOUR START DATE

Look at your calendar, see when you have time to do this, and commit. Successful goals are time-based and trackable. Ideally pick a 3-week window with minimal travel or family events. But the truth is, there is never a "perfect" time. There will always be a birthday or a business trip, so just choose the *best* time to start...in the not-too-distant future.

FAMILIARIZE YOURSELF WITH THE FOOD LISTS

See Chapter 5 for the full list.

ALLOWED FOODS

Below are all the mouthwatering foods that are allowed. We've divided the allowed foods into three categories:

◆ *"Totally Allowed"* (like vegetables and healthy proteins)

◆ *"Allowed in Moderation"* (whole wheat and whole grains, bread, pasta, fruit, healthy fats, and dairy)

◆ *"Barely Allowed"* (fattier proteins and higher calorie foods such as bacon, sausage, and french fries).

FOODS

These are the foods you can eat on the program, broken down into 3 categories to help you make the best choices.

TOTALLY ALLOWED

→ **Healthy proteins**
- Poultry
- Fish and shellfish
- Beef
- Eggs
- Tofu and tempeh
- Openfit Plant-Based Protein Shakes

→ **Beans and legumes**

→ **Vegetables**
- Lettuce and greens
- Carrots, tomatoes, cucumbers, etc.
- Broccoli, cauliflower, etc.

→ **Unsweetened flavor enhancers**
- Lemon
- Lime
- Salt and pepper
- Mustard
- Vinegar
- NSA ketchup

→ **Water, coffee, tea**

ALLOWED IN MODERATION

→ **Starchy vegetables**
- Potatoes
- Corn
- Winter squash

→ **Whole fruit**
- Apples
- Berries
- Bananas

→ **Unrefined whole grains**

→ **Approved whole grain breads and pasta**

→ **Healthy fats**
- Avocado
- Oils
- Nuts and nut butters

ALLOWED Foods

NOT ALLOWED FOODS

Here's where you'll find added sugars and foods with refined carbs and artificial sweeteners sneakily slipped in. I know it's tempting to want to push a button when you see the DO NOT PUSH BUTTON sign. (Why is that anyway?) But if you've read this far, you've heard my case about why added sugar and certain artificial sweeteners are detrimental to your health. Read the list, know thy enemy, and stay away.

{
*Be sure to check out the ALLOWED
and NOT ALLOWED FOODS
videos at Openfit.com/SF3 for more on this.*
}

FOODS

ALLOWED Foods

ALLOWED IN MODERATION continued

→ Full-fat and reduced-fat dairy

→ NSA milks

→ Stevia and monk fruit

- -

BARELY ALLOWED

→ High-fat proteins
- Bacon
- Sausage

→ Fried and high-fat foods
- French fries
- Potato chips
- Tortilla chips

NOT ALLOWED Foods

Added Sugars, Refined Carbs, and Artificial Sweeteners are not allowed for the next 21 days.

→ **Sugar and Other Sweet Things**
- Sugar, brown sugar, honey, agave, maple syrup, high fructose corn syrup
- Cookies, candy, and chocolate
- Ice cream and frozen yogurt
- Dried fruit with added sugar
- Soda, sweet tea, fruit juice

→ **Refined, Enriched, or White Flour Products**
- Bagels, English muffins, pitas, cereals, etc.
- Crackers, pretzels
- White rice and pasta
- Wine, beer, hard liquor

→ **Artificial Sweeteners and Products**
- Sucralose aka Splenda
- Aspartame aka Equal
- Saccharin aka Sweet'n Low
- Diet soda
- Sugar alcohols
- Sugarless gum and candy

Mindful Indulgence	Once a week, you may enjoy a food or beverage from the Not Allowed list *(it's optional but there if you need it).*
Exercise	Exercise is not required on **Sugar Free 3** but will boost the benefits. You'll find over 350 awesome workouts on Openfit.

LEARN HOW TO READ A FOOD LABEL

As discussed in Chapter 2, food manufacturers hide sugar in products you'd never expect in order to make them more appetizing, like bread and tomato sauce. So it's super important to learn how to read a food label so that you can definitively determine which foods (and beverages) are **SF3** approved. To help make it easier, I've created step-by-step instructions on how to read a food label. One critical thing to realize is that you're not *just* looking for grams of sugar on the nutrition panel—it's also about spotting the sneaky-sugar ingredients from the Sugar AKAs (see page 43).

◆ *Step A:* Pick up package—acknowledge the package and marketing and then turn over!

◆ *Step B:* Look for the ingredient list. Typically it's below the Nutrition Facts. Look for sugar, honey, high fructose corn syrup, or anything on the Sugar AKA list. Next, make sure all the grains are "whole" grains. Just the word "wheat" doesn't mean anything. Lastly you're looking for artificial sweeteners like aspartame, sucralose, or saccharin. If you see any of these ingredients, put the package back. If not, on to Step C!

◆ *Step C:* Go to the Nutrition Facts panel. Under Total Carbohydrate, look for the words Sugars or Added Sugars. You may not see "Added Sugars" yet but new labels laws will be requiring it soon. If you see Added Sugars, put the package down. Keep in mind, just because a product may have 6 grams of "Sugar" that doesn't mean it's not approved. Many foods have natural sugars and are Approved.

On following page you'll see approved and not approved labels as examples. If you're still confused, be sure to check out my reading label videos with registered dietitian Keri Glassman.

How to Read a Food Label

It just takes a moment to implement three simple steps.

YOU MAY FIND that a label has 0 grams of added sugars, but under the line sugar, you see 4 or 6 or even 8 grams. For example, see the label below for an **SF3**-approved plain Greek yogurt. The ingredient list looks good—there's no added sugars—and yet 5 grams of sugar. These are naturally occurring sugars, which makes this yogurt approved.

On the other hand, next to that we have a yogurt label that had added sugars and is therefore not approved:

APPROVED

Nutrition Facts

About 3 servings per container

Serving size	3/4 cup (170g)

Amount per serving

Calories **120**

% Daily Value*

Total Fat	3.5 g
Saturated Fat	2.5 g
Trans Fat	0 g
Cholesterol	20 mg
Sodium	55 mg
Total Carbohydrate	5 g
Dietary Fiber	0 g
Total Sugars	5 g
Incl. Added Sugars	0 g
Protein	17 g

Vit. D 0mcg 15%	Calcium 200mg 15%
Iron 0mg 0%	Potassium 260mg 6%

*The % Daily Values tells you how much a nutrient in a serving of food contributes to a daily diet. 2,000 calories a day is used for general nutrition advice.

*Product formulation and packaging may change. Plese refer to the product label for the most accurate information.

Ingredients: Grade A Pasteurized Skimmed Milk and Cream, Live Active Yogurt Cultures (L. Bulgaricus, S. Thermophilus, L. Acidophilus, Bifidus, L. Casei).

NOT APPROVED

Nutrition Facts

About 5 servings per container

Serving size	2/3 cup (170g)

Amount per serving

Calories **150**

% Daily Value*

Total Fat	1 g
Saturated Fat	0.5 g
Trans Fat	0 g
Cholesterol	<5 mg
Sodium	80 mg
Total Carbohydrate	31 g
Dietary Fiber	0 g
Total Sugars	22 g
Incl. Added Sugars	17 g
Protein	5 g

Vit. D 3.6mcg 15%	Calcium 180mg 15%
Iron 0mg 0%	Vitamin A 170mcg 15%

Potassium 240mg 6%

*Percent Daily Values are based on a 2,000 calorie diet. Your daily values may be higher or lower depending on your calorie needs.

Ingredients: Cultured Pasteurized Grade A Low Fat Milk, Sugar, Modified Corn Starch, Contains less than 1% of: Modified Tapioca [...]cid, Vegetable Juice (for color), [...]otassium Sorbate Added [...]ness, Vitamin A Acetate,

Step C: Look for "Added Sugars."

Step B: Look for anything on the Sugar AKA list in the ingredients.

For a comprehensive list of sugars hiding under secret identities, go to the Appendix.

Sugar AKAs

ONCE THE SUGAR industry realized it was busted on its fat-scare tactics and false "healthy" labels, it came up with a new way to smuggle this cheap and dangerous ingredient into our foods—right under our noses. "Yes, sugar hides in plain view," says Dr. Whitney Bowe. "Apart from the obvious places, if you look on a label you'll find it in unlikely places, such as hamburger buns, French fries, potato chips, and processed meats. It may be called something other than 'sugar,'" she continues. "Cane sugar, sucrose, fructose, agave nectar, high fructose corn syrup—but sugar is sugar, no matter how you spell it. There are more than sixty names for sugar! And it can be hard to avoid if you don't make a conscious effort and know what to look for."

The FDA requires food manufacturers to have an ingredients list on each of their products. "The ingredient list on a food label is the listing of each ingredient in descending order of predominance," says the FDA, which also rules that food manufacturers must "always list the common or usual name for ingredients unless there is a regulation that provides for a different term."

Just as they did with packaging health claims, food manufacturers found a loophole in the FDA ingredient list guidelines, and they got pretty creative with the terms they used to identify sugar. By referring to sugar with different names, food manufacturers thought they could trick the general public into thinking their foods didn't have any added or refined sugars.

They also started using several different types of added sugars in foods. This allowed the manufacturers to use numerous confusing terms for sugar when identifying ingredients on one single label. It also made it more difficult for even the most savvy label reader to estimate the ratio of added sugars and naturally occurring sugar in a product.

When you add them up, there are more than sixty names for sugar used on ingredient labels. Some of the most common sugar AKAs used by food manufacturers include the following:

AGAVE NECTAR

ARTIFICIAL SWEETENERS

- Aspartame
- Sucralose
- Saccharin

BARLEY MALT

BLACKSTRAP MOLASSES

BROWN RICE SYRUP

BROWN SUGAR

BUTTERED SYRUP

CANE JUICE CRYSTALS

CANE SUGAR

CARAMEL

CAROB SYRUP

CASTOR SUGAR

COCONUT SUGAR

CONFECTIONER'S SUGAR

CORN SYRUP

CORN SYRUP SOLIDS

DATE SUGAR

DEMERARA SUGAR

DEXTRIN

DEXTROSE

DIASTATIC MALT

ETHYL MALTOL

EVAPORATED CANE JUICE

FLORIDA CRYSTALS

FRUIT JUICE

FRUIT JUICE CONCENTRATE

FRUCTOSE

GLUCOSE

GLUCOSE SOLIDS

GOLDEN SUGAR

GOLDEN SYRUP

GRAPE SUGAR

HIGH FRUCTOSE CORN SYRUP

HONEY

ICING SUGAR

INVERT SUGAR

MALT SYRUP

MALTODEXTRIN

MALTOSE

MAPLE SYRUP

MOLASSES

MUSCOVADO SUGAR

PANELA SUGAR

RAW SUGAR

REFINER'S SYRUP

RICE SYRUP

SORGHUM SYRUP

SUCANAT

TREACLE SUGAR

TURBINADO SUGAR

UNREFINED SUGAR

YELLOW SUGAR

*For a complete list of alternate names for added sugars
and artificial sweeteners, see the Appendix.*

GET SET

Get Your Kitchen Ready

It's clean-out time. Go through your fridge, pantry, kitchen cabinets (and maybe your desk drawers or locker at work) and purge sugar, soda, candy, sweets, artificial sweeteners, and refined carbs, like bread and pretzels—anything that may tempt you. Why make this harder than it has to be?

Decide How You'll Do the Food

We're all different when it comes to food and eating. Whether you're a passionate home cook or never set foot in the kitchen and order take-out (or dine out) every night of the week, this plan will work for you. Here are three ways to organize your eating, which you can mix and match as needed.

- *LIKE TO COOK:* Pick this route if you love to food shop, meal prep, and cook. We've laid out a 7-day meal plan on page 113 along with a bunch of amazing, easy-to-make recipes to help get you started. Note: For your full 21-day meal plan, go to Openfit.com/**SF3**.

- *WILLING TO COOK:* This route is for those of you who don't have any desire to cook or don't have interest or time to spend in the kitchen. We've created a simpler way to follow the program with minimal shopping and prep work using pre-cut and washed veggies and even pre-cooked proteins. Refer to page 144 for more details.

- *DON'T COOK:* This route is specifically designed for those who are not into shopping, meal prepping, or cooking and will be taking out, ordering in or dining out. Just refer to page 158 the dining out guide in Chapter 7 to help navigate your choices.

Join the Sugar Free 3 Community

Download the Openfit app. We are all here to help you crush this! Adopting a new, healthy lifestyle is so much easier when you feel like you're part of a community—it keeps you accountable, you can get quick answers and support for any challenges you face, and you can share recipes, food finds, and other tips for taking the program to the next level. And yeah—why not show off a bit! We want to see and hear about the successes you've had with **Sugar Free 3**. And if you have questions, we're here to help.

Select a Sugar Sponsor

I highly recommend you designate someone who can support you during the next three weeks—whether that's your significant other, co-worker, friend, or family member. In fact you should tell everyone you know that you are doing **Sugar Free 3**, and maybe get some friends on board to do the program too!

GO!

Plan Your Meals

Now that you know how to put the program into action, start planning your **Sugar Free 3** meals. Whichever route you choose, I recommend you do a little forward thinking—even just a week at a time—to determine where you'll be eating or what you'll be cooking. Meal planning takes some time and organization, but it's a powerful tool for healthier eating and weight loss. And I always suggest that you strive for two things: first is balance in your meals, meaning protein, veggies, and a healthy carb and fat at each meal to keep your energy and cravings stable. The second is to keep it simple so you can stay consistent; I eat eggs, greens, and avocado (and some days toast) on most mornings; salads with quinoa for lunch; veggies and grilled protein and a healthy grain for dinner, spruced up with my favorite seasonings, of course.

At the end of the chapter you'll find some meal inspiration, and Chapter 5 provides a 7-day sample of the Like to Cook, Willing to Cook and Don't Cook plans.

And for a fully customized 21-day meal plan and meal and dining out ideas, go to Openfit.com/SF3.

Make a Weekly Grocery List and Go Shopping

Thanks to our increasingly busy schedules—and the all too accommodating rise of online food delivery—grocery shopping has evolved from a planned weekly ritual to an improvisational, as-needed activity. Nothing against having an extra hand sometimes, but this approach to grocery shopping can lead to unhealthy eating. Unfortunately, many of us (myself included) have come to view food shopping as a chore, instead of a strategic play that can benefit your health and help you reach your goals. So now that you have your meals planned, it's easy to make a grocery list of what foods you need for the week before you hit the grocery store. Going to the store with a list will help keep you focused and help you avoid those snacks and foods you don't need. (Bonus: It'll probably save you money, too.)

GROCERY SHOPPING GUIDE

A few tips before you fill your cart...

▶ *Always start with the perimeter of the supermarket.* That's where the mainstays of your meals will be located. You'll notice fruits and vegetables, healthy proteins, and low-fat dairy are mostly in the outer aisles.

▶ *Avoid anything on the NOT ALLOWED List.* Usually in the inner aisles.

▶ *Load up on veggies and fresh produce.* Not to be confused with "taste the rainbow" (the candy slogan, which you definitely shouldn't follow), "eat the rainbow" is nutritionists' credo, which you definitely should adhere to. Adding a full spectrum of colorful fruits and vegetables to your diet is a shortcut to total nutrition, overall health, and weight loss. In Chapter 5, we'll talk more about the benefits of colorful vegetables you should eat in abundance.

▶ *Find healthy proteins.* You have permission to go a little crazy here. Fill your basket with as many sources of healthy protein—chicken, fish, eggs, lean beef, turkey, pork, and tofu—as you like. Protein keeps you fuller for longer, and it helps to preserve fat-burning lean muscle, whether you regularly hit the gym or not.

▶ *Don't snub healthy fats.* Remember: The message that all fats are bad is an eighties relic that should never be revived. (Madonna and puff-sleeve sweaters: Yes. Fat-free diets: No.) Healthy fats—such as those found in olive oil, avocados, nuts, seeds, and cold-water fish like salmon—are absolutely key to a healthy diet. They keep you satiated (meaning you'll be less likely to crave sugary, simple carbs between meals) and have been associated with heart and brain health.

▶ *Seek out no-sugar-added flavor boosters.* As you'll see in the next chapter, there are a plethora of seasonings that can add a ton of flavor to your meals with minimal calories. Many have heart-healthy, metabolism-stoking benefits of their own. We're talking mustard, hot sauce, vinegar, lemon, lime, fresh salsa, fresh and dried herbs and spices, sea salt, pepper, and blends like Everything But the Bagel seasoning (a personal fave). You'll see that a little goes a long way toward making your meals delicious and satisfying.

▶ *Stock up on the recommended staples,* so you don't find yourself facing bare cupboards—the ultimate nemesis. Knowing you have Greek yogurt and fresh strawberries in the fridge or frozen grapes (one of my go-tos) for a snack can help you resist the temptation to pick up a half-gallon of ice cream. When you're exhausted from a day of meetings or a long shift, realizing you have the fixings for Grilled Chicken Paillard with Red Wine Vinaigrette at home (or better yet, pre-prepared!) makes it not just easy, but attractive, to bypass your usual drive-through on the way home.

▶ *Read labels to spot added sugars.* You now know sugar is hiding everywhere. So always check the ingredients list and the Nutrition Facts panel. (Reminder: Bring your reading glasses to the supermarket, if you need them!)

Document Your Day 1

It may sound silly, but take a full-body selfie (in a bathing suit, if possible) and also a closeup of your face, which often shows the first signs of weight loss, not to mention you'll notice your skin get glowier. Don't worry, you never have to share it, if you don't want to. I also recommend you weigh yourself, especially if one of your goals is weight loss. Trust me, on day 21 you'll be psyched to look back to see how far you've come! START EATING!

YUMMY MEAL INSPIRATION

W HEN OUR TEST groups tried **Sugar Free 3**, they were psyched about how much food they were allowed to eat. In Chapter 5, you'll find more than 40 satisfying recipes you can make at home. I put together a few quick ideas here, so you can get a sense of how simple it is to do this for three weeks. For optimal energy, I recommend that you strive for balance at meal time and select a balance of veggies, healthy protein, healthy carbs, and healthy fat to fill your plate or bowl.

BREAKFAST

▶ *Idea 1:* Eggs, greens, avocado, and salsa. (It's optional, but you could add a little sweet potato, fruit or **SF3**-approved toast.)

▶ *Idea 2:* Greek yogurt with a tablespoon of nut butter or 2 table-spoons of peanut butter powder and berries.

▶ *Idea 3:* Avocado toast made with **SF3**-approved whole grain bread, and an egg (prepared however you prefer).

LUNCH

▶ *Idea 1:* Salad with grilled shrimp, veggies, sliced avocado, oil and vinegar, or NSA dressing. (Optional: add brown rice or black beans.)

▶ *Idea 2:* A healthy bowl made of mixed veggies, grilled salmon and avocado. (Optional: add quinoa or brown rice—or a mix of the two!)

▶ *Idea 3:* Grilled chicken cutlet with greens, cherry tomatoes, fresh herbs, and a drizzle of extra-virgin olive oil. (Optional: add an allow-able whole grain.)

DINNERS

▶ *Idea 1:* Grilled steak and sautéed spinach. (Optional: add a baked potato with Greek yogurt as a sour cream substitute.)

▶ *Idea 2:* Any type of lean protein and veggies, drizzle with healthy oil. (Optional: add baked "fries" or **SF3**-approved bun.)

▶ *Idea 3:* Broiled fish, roasted asparagus, mushrooms, and cauliflower. (Optional: brown rice or quinoa.)

SNACKS

▶ A piece of whole fruit (like a peach) or a cup of blueberries with plain Greek yogurt.

▶ Two hard-boiled eggs, with salt or other seasoning.

▶ Roasted sweet potato wedges with a drizzle of coconut oil.

▶ Raw veggies (jicama, cucumbers, and celery are good) and guacamole.

▶ Green apple with nut butter.

▶ Air-popped popcorn sprinkled with cumin, cinnamon, or cayenne.

▶ Mary's Gone Crackers with hummus.

{
Want The Best Results Possible?

Go to OPENFIT.COM/SF3 to access

my exclusive videos, recipes, 21-day customized

meal plan, food tracking and more.
}

Hooray! You Get a Mindful Indulgence

I DON'T KNOW ABOUT you, but when someone says I can't have something, I tend to fixate on it. That's why when we were developing the program we decided to include what I call a Mindful Indulgence. Once a week you get to mindfully (key word) indulge in something on the Not Allowed list—whether that's a glass of wine (yes, please!) or a slice of pizza. But I want to stress this: The Mindful Indulgence is completely optional...you don't have to have it. The reason I included it? While testing **SF3**, we found that most participants liked the idea of knowing they could have a treat once a week, even if they didn't end up partaking. Looking forward to the Mindful Indulgence helped some stay tried and true to the program. But if you think a taste of sugar might just trigger you, then stay the course of being sugar free. I, for one, will give you major props for displaying that kind of willpower.

SECRETS OF SUCCESS
Real-Life Tips from Me and the Very First
Sugar Free 3 Success Stories!

▶ *Drink MORE water.* Water is your ally, sparkling or still, room temperature or over ice or with lemon or lime. Aim for half your body weight in ounces a day—even more if you're experiencing headaches or cravings.

▶ *Track your food, mood, and anything else.* Food tracking is proven to help people achieve their health and nutrition goals, and you'll be amazed at how the simple task of writing things down helps you to be more aware and mindful of what you eat, especially if weight loss is your goal. And it doesn't have to be fancy. Write in a notebook, get a simple food tracker, use the Openfit app, or even jot it in notes on your phone. Track the food you eat, your mood, sleep, daily challenges you overcame, snack discoveries, favorite meals, and more. If you slip, write it down and get back on track! (For more on mindfulness and journaling info or tips, see Chapter 8.).

▶ *Exercise.* Exercise is always recommended but not required on **Sugar Free 3**. That said, exercise is key to any healthy lifestyle—and it's a great distraction when you're having cravings. The Department of Health and Human Services recommends 150 minutes of moderate aerobic activity (like a brisk walk, swim, or—if you can believe it—mowing the lawn) or 75 minutes of vigorous aerobic activity (like a good run) a week. Do what you like. If that means a walk or a jog, enjoy. But if you're looking for something more exciting and varied, visit Openfit.com, where you'll find a wide variety of workouts—including a few created specifically to supplement the results of **Sugar Free 3**.

▶ *Hop on the scale for a weekly weigh-in.* Some people fear the scale, some people weigh themselves daily, but weekly weigh-ins are a good way to check in to see if you're on track toward your goals. Be sure to check Chapter 6, which is dedicated to weight loss.

▶ *Embrace the food-prep process.* A little planning and organization can go a long way so you can have control of what you eat and never be caught off guard. Whether it's your breakfast, lunch, or dinner, I highly recommended meal planning. As countless Instagrammers have shown, #mealprep can be a #delicious and #satisfying (even #artistic) Sunday routine. You can make a galaxy of variations on overnight oats or avocado toast for breakfast; hard-boiled egg or egg bites; beautiful lunch grain bowls replete with greens and protein; or envy-inspiring dinners of lean, savory chicken, fish, or beef. By the way, if you do decide to post your meal mastery on social, be sure to use the hashtag **#SugarFree3**.

▶ *Follow the program your way.* The best eating plans are flexible and adaptable to real life. **Sugar Free 3** is exactly that. If you're a meat-eater, you'll have plenty to choose from. The same goes if you're a vegetarian (tofu and tempeh). If you like to eat breakfast for dinner, be my guest. Mealtimes are up to you. **Sugar Free 3** isn't about regimenting *when* you eat, but is more about *what* you're eating. We recommend three meals a day, but again, you have to do it your way, so if you're an intermittent faster and like to skip breakfast, do it. We're excited to hear how you tweak things to suit your lifestyle.

▶ *Remember, it's just three weeks!* You can stay on the plan long-term, or you can revisit it after the holidays or a vacation when you've been overindulging and feel sluggish. (I find it resets my system.) For first-timers, all I'm asking for is three short weeks.

CHAPTER

4

THE FOOD LISTS

An In-Depth Look at What You'll Be Eating (and Ditching)

WHAT ARE THE scariest words in the English language? For some people it's *We need to talk.* For others it's *You might want to sit down for this.* For me, it's *You're not allowed to have that.* Specifically, these words strike fear in my heart when they are applied to eating. When I am told I can't have something, I just want it more! I'm not sure what that says about me, but it's true. I don't do deprivation well. So when I created **Sugar Free 3**, I knew that if I was going to ask you to avoid added sugars, desserts, refined bread and pasta, and diet soda, I had to replace them with options that were equally filling and satisfying, as if to say, "You can't have *that*, but look at all of *this*!"

So I worked with registered dietitians, professional chefs, and other nutrition experts to provide a bountiful list of proteins, healthy fats, delicious veggies, and carbs—yes, carbs!—that taste great together and are easy to procure and prepare to ensure that you will never feel hungry while on this plan.

The Allowed Foods in this chapter make up the core of **Sugar Free 3**. You'll see they're divided into three categories:

Totally Allowed. These foods are the mainstay of your program and should constitute the majority of what you eat during mealtimes and snacks. Now I won't tell you to eat *unlimited* amounts of anything, but it'll be hard to mess up by eating these foods. *(Be sure to check out the recipes later in the book starting on page 111.)*

Allowed in Moderation. These foods are added-sugar–free, but often higher in calories than foods on the Totally Allowed list. They can be enjoyed in moderation at every meal. And if weight loss is one of your goals, you should definitely not overindulge in these.

Barely Allowed. These foods are tasty and technically added-sugar–free, but they aren't the healthiest options—they're nutrition-poor and often packed with calories, unhealthy fats, and sodium. They are sanctioned on this plan, but we recommend limiting to 1–2 servings per day.

> ### What does NSA mean? *NSA stands for No Sugar Added, and you'll see this term pop up throughout the book. For example: "Be sure to check out our NSA marinara and ketchup which are fresher and better tasting than store-brought brands."*

TOTALLY ALLOWED

Healthy Proteins

CHICKEN AND TURKEY, FISH AND SHELLFISH, LEAN BEEF, LEAN PORK, EGGS, TOFU AND TEMPEH, BEANS AND LEGUMES

+ unsweetened protein powders such as pea, hemp, and casein or Openfit plant-based protein

SUPERPOWERS: Proteins are made of amino acids, the body's primary building blocks. They can also help with weight loss because they take longer to digest, making you feel fuller for longer so you won't be reaching for those extra munchies.

SECRET WEAPONS: Healthy protein-based foods are also loaded with tons of other nutrients, including selenium, B vitamins, vitamin D, iron, choline, zinc, magnesium, and omega 3 fatty acids (particularly in fatty fish).

POSERS: Fattier cuts of meat, ground beef that's less than 85 percent lean (including meatballs and meatloaf), hot dogs, sausage, bacon, and most other processed meats, which are all higher in either saturated fat or nasty additives and preservatives.

Every one of these healthy proteins helps you feel fuller longer, and has an astonishing number of benefits like building lean muscle mass, which means you burn more calories even when you're at rest. That'll make them your BFFs on this plan or any other.

Now that I've introduced you to these new pals, let's get to know them a little better.

Chicken and Turkey

Poultry, particularly skinless white meat, is a great source of lean protein, with iron, magnesium, and B vitamins, which are believed to help support your metabolism. Some of my favorite tips for buying and using poultry are:

Skinless Chicken Breasts. So versatile, these can be thrown into the oven with some EVOO and a few spices and then sliced for salads.

Ground. Ground turkey and chicken work really well for both burgers and meatballs. You'll find scrumptious recipes for these on the Openfit app.

Pre-Cooked Poultry. I buy it at the beginning of the week and have enough for a few days of dinners or lunches.

NSA, Nitrate-, and Nitrite-Free Deli Meat. A great and easy source of protein, especially on the go, but keep in mind they are typically packed with sodium, so look for low-sodium versions.

Fish and Shellfish

I have cultivated a love of seafood by spending summers at the Jersey shore. And I loved it even more after learning that many fish, especially some wild-caught cold-water fish, are packed with omega-3 essential fatty acids.

We need a balance of omega-3 and omega-6 fatty acids to thrive. Your diet is likely already filled with omega-6s (found in proteins like meat, poultry, and eggs, as well as soybeans, corn, certain oils, and nuts), so it's important to focus on anti-inflammatory omega-3s. There are a few kinds, and fish is a good source of two of them that the body absorbs readily: DHA and EPA. Salmon, Pacific oysters, sardines, anchovies, and herring are top picks, and all are packed full of omega-3 fatty acids. Additionally, the United States Department of Agriculture reported that consuming about 8 ounces of a variety of seafood per week can help prevent heart disease. (By the way, a fatty fish such as salmon isn't a lean protein because, obviously, it's fatty—but these are mostly healthy fats like omega-3s.)

How to decode labels:

Farm-Raised: These fish are raised in enclosed environments. Generally, they are thought of as less healthy, and I have definitely worried about whether I should eat them. My expert buds tell me that USA-based farm-raised tilapia, mussels, trout, and Arctic char are the smartest "farm-raised" options.

Wild-Caught: Swimming freely in oceans, rivers, lakes, or ponds, these fish have a more varied diet than farmed fish, and thus they tend to have a richer color and flavor.

Some notes about buying:

Fresh usually tastes better than frozen. But there's no health difference between the two.

Canned (or pouched) tuna or salmon works great for lunches or snacks because it's portable protein. Go for the kind in water to avoid unnecessary oils. If you're concerned about mercury, opt for light tuna or stick with salmon.

Pre-cooked will save you time in the kitchen, and it's great to toss into salads, stir-fry recipes, lettuce wraps, or to eat as a snack.

Some winners:

The Best Fish and Shellfish: Anchovies, black sea bass, Chilean sea bass, clams, cod, crab, crawfish, flounder, haddock, hake, halibut, herring, lobster, oysters, pollock, salmon (I prefer wild Alaskan over Atlantic), sardines, scallop, shrimp, skate, sole, squid, tilapia, trout, freshwater tuna (canned light, includes skipjack), whitefish, whiting—so many!

Smart to Avoid: If you're not pregnant and you're an adult, the consensus among most experts is that you don't need to stress about the mercury levels in fish too much. Still, I don't eat king mackerel, marlin, orange roughy, shark, swordfish, tilefish (from the Gulf of Mexico) or bigeye tuna, just in case.

Smokin'! *Maybe it's because I'm a New Yorker, but I love smoked salmon for breakfast (sans bagel on **Sugar Free 3**). Scramble it with eggs or enjoy it on **SF3**-approved toast. I'll even slice it up and mix it into a spinach salad for a hit of protein and salt. Plus, it keeps a long time in the refrigerator, and now you can find a whole bunch of delicious flavored varieties. (Note: Some types have added maple syrup or other sugars—so be sure to read the ingredients.)*

Lean Beef

It may have a bad reputation, but beef isn't the "red menace" it's been made out to be. For most people, a moderate amount of red meat a few times a week is totally fine. When buying beef, here are my tips.

Buyer Beware: *Stay away from processed meats and cured meats like hot dogs and bacon. Besides being high in saturated fat, salt, and cholesterol, some contain sugar, and sodium nitrates. Combined with amines, an organic compound found in the meat, nitrites can result in a potentially cancer-causing compound.*

THE BEST IN BEEF

Grass Fed is my go-to. I think it tastes better than grain-fed, and furthermore "grass fed meat is lower in total fat, which is really cool because there's less calories per nutrient. It's very a nutrient-dense food," says *Genius Foods* author Max Lugavere. "It's also a great source of minerals. It's generally more expensive, but I'm a firm believer that by paying more for health, and higher-quality groceries, you're going to save money down the road because if there's anything that's expensive, it's disease."

Organic Beef is also key because it means the animal never received growth hormones or antibiotics, wasn't genetically engineered, and was allowed continuous access to the outdoors per USDA guidelines.

Cuts above the Rest

▸ *Steaks.* Sirloin tip, tenderloin, top round, eye round, flank steak, top sirloin, and flap steak are among the leanest cuts of beef.

▸ *Ground.* Great for burgers and meatballs, when buying ground meat look for at least 85–90 percent lean.

Lean Pork

The fatty portion of the pork chop can account for about two thirds of the chop's fat content, so when opting for this "other white meat," go for lean pork over the pulled type or fried-up bacon. Tenderloin, boneless pork chop, top loin roast, and pork rib chop are good options.

Eggs

I'm obsessed with eggs, they're so damn good—and so versatile that you can eat them for any meal of the day. They're super-easy to cook (on the Openfit app, you'll find a ton of my favorite recipes). If you were raised to believe that egg yolks lead to a spare tire or muffin top, soaring

How good is "good"?

The Food and Drug Administration actually regulates words like "good" and "excellent" when it comes to describing food.

▶ If you see the words "good source," "contains," or "provides" on the package, that means a serving of that food contains 10 to 19 percent of the reference daily intake (RDI) or Daily Reference Value (DRV) for that nutrient.

▶ If you see the words "high," "rich in," or "excellent source of," that means a serving has 20 percent of more of the RDI or DRV for the nutrient.

▶ So if the label on those whole grain crackers you're snacking on says they "contain" iron, that means that they have 10 to 19 percent of the amount of iron most healthy people need each day.

cholesterol, and a stern warning from your doctor, take solace in this: Newer research suggests you might want to give eggs a break...open. Though the yolk has saturated fat and cholesterol (the sources of the controversy), it's also dense in nutrients like iron and other vitamins and minerals, and two carotenoids called lutein and zeaxanthin that keep your eyes healthy (the more of these two in a yolk, the deeper the color). The choline in yolks is good for brain health. Unless your doctor tells you otherwise, most experts agree that one egg a day, on average, is good. Have another if you're not worried about cholesterol.

Egg whites are basically pure protein. There's not much in terms of other nutrients, but if you're just looking to add a muscle-builder to your day, the white is the way. Here's a quick glossary of the eggs you'll find in stores. Different certifiers have different requirements, but here are some general guidelines:

Caged. You won't see this term on your egg carton—what company would want to promote it?! But unless you see one of the phrases below, assume the eggs were produced by hens confined to cages.

Cage-Free. The hens aren't kept in cages, but they aren't allowed outside of a barn or henhouse.

Free-Range. This means the hens are allowed outside, but their yard isn't huge and may not be required to contain vegetation.

Pastured. Not only are these hens allowed outside, but they roam free in a natural pasture where they can eat the seeds and bugs they were born to eat. They really do taste "farm-fresh." What's more, researchers at Penn State found that, compared to eggs from hens getting commercial feed, eggs from pasture-raised hens also had twice as much vitamin E and more than double the total omega-3 fatty acids.

EGG-CELLENT TIPS

▶ Look for egg whites in a carton in the fridge section

▶ Grab pre-cooked eggs to save time

▶ Save fat and calories by poaching or hard-boiling

Tofu and Tempeh

Tofu may feel like a seventies health food store staple, but it is suddenly on every salad menu now that plant-based proteins and vegan lifestyles are so popular, and for good reason: It's a terrific source of calcium and even some omega-3s. Tempeh is a fermented soy product that has a meaty, tender bite with a semi-nutty flavor. It will absorb any flavor, and a standard 3-ounce serving has about 16 grams of protein and 8 percent of the day's recommended calcium.

Whenever possible, purchase organic varieties. That also makes it non-GMO, which means you'll avoid herbicides and other chemicals. Additionally, other plant-based foods like beans, lentils, nuts, seeds (e.g., chia and hemp), and whole grains like quinoa and buckwheat are also great sources of protein. You'll learn more about them later in this chapter.

Is Soy OK for Guys? *Soy contains estrogen-like chemicals called phytoestrogens, but a guy would have to consume an insane amount before he'd need to worry about growing man-boobs. In moderation, everyone can incorporate soy foods—unsweetened soy milk, edamame, tofu—several times per week without an impact on testosterone levels.*

Beans and Legumes

Chickpeas and Hummus, Lentils, Fava Beans, Black Beans, Green Peas

+ canned baked beans without added sugars, dried chickpeas, edamame, bean pasta, and other beans with minimal to no salt

SUPERPOWERS: A trifecta of protein, fiber, and steady-energy carbs.

SECRET WEAPONS: B vitamins, fiber, iron, folate, zinc, calcium, copper, phosphorus, potassium, manganese.

POSERS: Refried beans (the traditional kind with lard); baked beans with added sugars, fat, and salt; most bean-based chips or other "crispy" bagged snacks.

Thanks to the highly-processed modern American diet, the average American isn't getting enough of one of the most important nutrients: fiber. Without a consistent intake of healthy soluble and insoluble high-fiber foods in your diet, you'll experience dips in energy, have difficulty losing weight, and risk constipation.

Enter beans and legumes.

Lentils, black beans, white beans, chickpeas, fava beans, kidney beans, pinto beans, black-eyed peas, soybeans—every bean but jelly beans has benefits.

Versatile and affordable, beans help keep the gut clean, and they also help you lose weight. The *American Journal of Clinical Nutrition* reported that people who added just a ¾-cup serving of beans, peas, chickpeas, or lentils also felt 31 percent fuller, which may have contributed to weight loss.

One Note

Beans, in particular, contain oligosaccharides. The body doesn't break down this naturally occurring carbohydrate completely at first, which results in flatulence. But don't despair. There are a few ways to prevent yourself from sounding like the horn section of the band post–bean consumption.

▶ Soak and rinse beans well before prepping.

▶ Cook until soft.

▶ Try a digestive enzyme supplement. My favorites are Enzymedica and Pure Synergy Enzyme Power, but Beano may be the easiest to find.

▶ Don't scarf them down. Chew and eat them slowly.

▶ Add them into your diet gradually.

USE YOUR BEAN!

▶ Make beans your main or side dish, and incorporate them into soups, salads, chili, or pasta dishes.

▶ Eat them mashed in homemade or store-bought spreads and dips like hummus.

▶ Explore bean pastas; just be sure to check the ingredient list to make sure the only ingredient is beans (no added flour).

▶ For canned beans, purchase the low-sodium or no-sodium varieties, and rinse before eating.

Why Fiber is Your Friend

IT KEEPS YOU full and fit, so why is fiber's vibe uncool? Probably because it's typically associated with curing bathroom-related challenges. So let's recast fiber in a more positive light. After all, it is an essential building block in a healthy lifestyle and, if consumed properly, can actually relieve discomfort and bloating. Yay, fiber!

Fiber 101

▶ *Dietary Fiber:* A class of complex carbohydrates described as an indigestible long chain of sugar molecules. It is naturally found in complex carb foods such as fruits, veggies, grains, and legumes. Fiber is a class of carbohydrates that can be further broken down into two different forms: soluble and insoluble.

▶ *Soluble Fiber:* This fiber combines with water to form a gel-like substance that creates bulk. This gel-like fiber helps to slow digestion, keeping you fuller longer and helping to maintain healthy blood sugar levels. Soluble fiber is also the type of fiber known for boosting heart health. Chia seeds, for example, are particularly rich in soluble fiber. Other examples include oatmeal and oat bran, beans, and nuts.

▶ *Insoluble Fiber:* Rather than dissolve in water, insoluble fiber moves through your digestive tract undigested. This bulking feature of insoluble fiber helps to move food through your body, adding bulk to stool. You'll find insoluble fiber in seeds, whole wheat, brown rice, and fruit and veggie skins. (I'm not asking you to eat bananas whole, but you really shouldn't peel apples.)

Your Daily Fiber Intake

Americans should consume at least 28 grams of fiber per day if they're following a 2,000 calorie diet, according to the FDA.

Unfortunately, we're getting nowhere close to that amount. A report from the Food and Drug Administration says that the average American woman eats only 15 grams of fiber a day, while the average adult man consumes just under 19 grams per day. The problem is likely due to us being confused about what's good and what's bad. Here's a handy reference:

- *Fiber Full*
  Fresh fruit (with the peel on)
  Fresh vegetables
  Whole grain bread
  Brown rice
  Popcorn

- *Fiber Less*
  Fruit juice
  Most green juice
  White bread
  White rice

And when it comes to packaged foods, always look for "excellent" sources instead of "good" ones. This one swap means you'll potentially double your fiber intake from 2.8 grams to 5.6 grams per serving.

Bean There, Done That Snacks

N EED A SNACK? Carry around a pack of some dried chickpeas or edamame.

Naturally nutty, fibrous, and filling, they have pops of flavor and zero sugar. Some options are below. Be sure to only grab the *Sea Salt* flavors, as other varieties, like Wasabi or Sriracha, have added sugars:

- ▶ *Biena Chickpea Snacks* Great when you're craving something salty and crunchy like chips. They're made with three simple ingredients that you can actually pronounce— chickpeas, sunflower oil, and sea salt—and have 6 grams of protein per serving.

- ▶ *Seapoint Farms Dry Roasted Edamame* Now you can carry your favorite sushi restaurant appetizer with you—in crispy form.

- ▶ *Bada Bean Bada Boom* Lightly salted dried broad beans— aka fava beans—in grab-and-go bags. They have more fiber and protein, and less fat, than even almonds.

Vegetables

Asparagus, Broccoli, Brussels Sprouts, Cabbage, Carrots, Cauliflower, Cucumbers, Mushrooms, Peppers, Lettuce and Leafy Greens, Spinach, Tomato, and NSA Pickled and Fermented Veggies

SUPERPOWERS: Low in fat and calories, high in important dietary fiber, helps keep your heart healthy.

SECRET WEAPONS: Vitamins A, C, E, and K, and carotenoids and other antioxidants, fiber, B vitamins, potassium, folate, lutein and—surprise!—even some protein!

POSERS: Stay away from canned veggies soaked in salt and those fried or drenched in cheese or butter; veggie-based "potato" chips, puffs, or other salt-filled bagged snacks, some cauliflower crusts and products, processed "veggie" dips (mix up a dip from scratch!).

Vegetables offer a rainbow—literally—of nutrition. In fact, phytonutrients, plant-based compounds that make veggies (and fruits) so healthy, also provide their distinct colors. So let's break them down by hue.

Green

What to eat: *spinach, broccoli, asparagus, kale, romaine lettuce, chard and other leafy greens, cucumber, zucchini*

Phytonutrients: *chlorophyll, lutein, zeaxanthin, indoles, isothiocyanate, flavonoids, and sulforaphane*

My approach to leafy greens is simple: The ones I absolutely love, like a spicy arugula and mixed lettuces, I eat raw in salads. Heartier ones, such as kale, escarole, or even spinach, I steam or sauté with some EVOO and garlic.

Red

What to eat: *beets, red carrots, peppers, tomatoes, radishes, cabbage*
Phytonutrients: *lycopene, ellagic acid, hesperidin, and anthocyanin*

When I think of red foods, I think of my favorite dishes: caprese salad or this radish app served with butter and salt at one of my favorite places; a classic beet and goat cheese salad with walnuts; red peppers in a soft chicken taco. All of those dishes are allowed on **Sugar Free 3**.

Orange and Yellow

What to eat: *carrots, peppers, golden beets, yellow squash, and spaghetti squash*
Phytonutrients: *beta-carotene, alpha-carotenoids, hesperetin, beta-cryptoxanthin, and lutein*

Not only do chopped-up yellow and orange veggies add oft-needed dramatic flair to any leafy green salad, but they tend to contain plenty of beta-carotene, an important phytonutrient that your body converts to vitamin A.

White

What to eat: *cauliflower, cabbage, mushrooms, onions, turnips, garlic, ginger*
Phytonutrients: *anthoxanthins, allicin*

Just because a veggie isn't bursting with color doesn't mean it's unworthy. For example, there's high amounts of vitamins C and B and about 3.5 grams of fiber in one cup of cooked cauliflower. It also beautifully absorbs the flavors you send its way—cheese, spices—and can be transformed into a plethora of different textures. Who knew one plant could have so many personalities?

Cauli-Madness!

WHO NEEDS REFINED carbs when you can have cauliflower? The vegetable once thought of as "broccoli's more boring lookalike" is having a big moment, quickly replacing all your favorite everything—hot cereals, crackers, chips, hash browns, bread, pizza crust—and tastes just as good, when done right. Be sure to read the labels to check for added flour and sugars. I love:

OUTER AISLE PLANTPOWER SANDWICH THINS
A too-good-to-be-true bread substitute, made with just fresh cauliflower, whole cage-free eggs, Parmesan cheese, and pure nutritional yeast.

GREEN GIANT OR TRADER JOE CAULIFLOWER RICE—FRESH AND FROZEN
An alternative to rice for a stir-fry or even to throw into your shakes; higher in fiber too. Be sure to read labels to make sure cauliflower is the only ingredient.

CALI'FLOUR FOODS PIZZA CRUST
Cauliflower pizza crusts are everywhere; this one has zero sugar added and only 90 calories per serving. Mangia!

MAKE THIS!
Try mashed cauliflower (even with garlic) and anything else you would do with traditional potatoes.

VEGGIE TIPS

▶ When purchasing produce, buy fresh if you can, but flash-frozen veggies also work as the flash freezing process retains the valuable nutrients.

▶ Look for no-salt-added canned vegetables if you like to keep your cabinets stocked.

▶ When preparing veggies, steam, bake, roast or grill if possible to keep in all those great nutrients. Boiling isn't a great option since it can leach out nutrients, including potassium and magnesium.

Unsweetened Flavor Enhancers

Mustard, NSA Hot Sauce, Vinegar,
Fresh-Squeezed Lemon and Lime,
Fresh Salsa and Pico de Gallo, Herbs and Spices,
Sea Salt, Horseradish, Pepper, Spice Mixes

SUPERPOWERS: Turns boring healthy food into exciting healthy food! Low in calories, but packed with flavor, these are all-you-can-eat!

SECRET WEAPONS: Lycopene, vitamins A, C, and E, selenium, magnesium, capsaicin, antioxidants.

POSERS: Ketchup, barbecue, Worcestershire and teriyaki sauce, sugar-added hot sauces (often manufactured with high fructose corn syrup), sweet chili sauce, cocktail sauce, most jams, jellies, and syrups and most bottled salad dressings.

Mustard

Whether it's Dijon, spicy brown, seeded, or good old yellow, mustard is the ultimate flavor enhancer. Just make sure to read the ingredients list. All you want to see is mustard seed, vinegar, salt, and water. (Be especially careful that they don't sneak any sugar in there.)

NSA Hot Sauce

The secret here: capsaicin. Chili peppers in hot sauce are high in this antioxidant-like substance that is believed to be linked to revving up the metabolism and weight loss.

Vinegar

The easy way to add zing to everything from salad to soup. Enjoy red wine, white, apple cider. Beware of balsamic because it contains "grape must," which is basically the same thing as grape juice, and definitely avoid balsamic glazes as they have added sugar.

Fresh-Squeezed Lemon and Lime

Since one lemon contains about half of your daily recommended amount of vitamin C, stocking up on the citrus fruit will make you immortal... or at least look like you are.

And let's not forget about lemon's "other half." Lime is high in antioxidants, especially vitamin C.

Fresh Salsa and Pico de Gallo

To make your own, just throw tomatoes, onions, cilantro, chili peppers, and a little salt into a food processor. Grind it up to the desired consistency. If you buy it in the store—I know I'm starting to sound like a broken record—check the ingredients to make sure there are no added sugars, but you're safe with most brands.

Herbs and Spices

Whether dried or fresh, spices and herbs can replace sugar and reduce salt, they add so much flavor. I've put together a list of ones you probably have on your shelf and what I pair them with:

Basil—pork, lamb, fish, cucumbers, tomatoes

Oregano—beef, pork, lamb, fish, green beans, eggplant, tomatoes

Dill—beef, lamb, poultry, fish, green beans, carrots, cucumbers, potatoes, eggs

Parsley—beef, pork, poultry, fish, carrots, cucumbers, eggplant

Rosemary—beef, pork, lamb, carrots, potatoes

Curry—beef, pork, lamb, poultry, fish, fruit

Mint—beef, poultry, lamb, fruit, veggies

Nutmeg—poultry, fish, fruit, green beans, beets, broccoli, carrots, squash

Chives—fish, potatoes

Fennel—fish, potatoes, tomatoes

Tarragon—corn, eggs, salmon, chicken, asparagus

Sage—beef, chicken, pork, whole grain pasta

Have fun experimenting. I love to mix basil, tarragon, and parsley into my scrambled eggs. A big hit with early adopters of **SF3** was Everything But the Bagel Sesame Blend from Trader Joe's.

WHAT CAN I DRINK?

Unsweetened Beverages

WATER, COFFEE, TEA, SELTZER, CLUB SODA

SUPERPOWERS: Hydration, flushes out the system.

SECRET WEAPONS: Antioxidants (coffee, tea).

POSERS: Sweetened tea and coffee, anything ending in "-chino," fruit juices, sports drinks (electrolyte-infused sugar water), soda (the "s-word").

We are water—it makes up 60 percent of our body and 90 percent of our blood—and it is essential for proper kidney function, flushes waste out of our bodies, helps deliver oxygen throughout the body, regulates body temperature, and more.

Also, water may help to fill your tummy, and being dehydrated is potentially linked to a slower metabolism.

Drink half your body weight in ounces every day; more if you're experiencing strong cravings, headaches, or work out often. Here's how to keep it fresh:

◆ Carbonated water (e.g., seltzer, sparkling water) is a fine alternative to the still stuff. Flavored seltzers for the most part are great. Just read the label to make sure there are no calories, no added sugars, or artificial sweeteners.

◆ Packed with natural antioxidants, black coffee is looking more and more like a health elixir in the eyes of modern science, and the natural caffeine gives your system a natural boost—mentally and physically. I take mine with a little milk and stevia.

◆ A cup of herbal tea is part of my nightly wind-down—I do ginger, lemon, licorice, or peppermint. Think outside of the bag:

    Muddle it—Mash up mint leaves and lime with a muddler and add cold water.

    Make ice cubes—Pour tea into an ice tray and savor on a hot day.

    Try loose leaf—The step-by-step process of filling a tea infuser adds a mindful moment to an already relaxing ritual.

If you're looking for milk, you'll find it under the Allowed in Moderation category, since I generally recommend you avoid drinking your calories.

ALLOWED IN MODERATION

These foods are blissfully allowed, but please eat them in moderation because they're higher in calories and carbs. If your goal is weight loss, we recommend no more than 3–4 servings a day.

Starchy Veggies

POTATOES; SWEET POTATOES; CORN; PUMPKIN, BUTTERNUT, ACORN, KABOCHA, AND OTHER WINTER SQUASH; CASSAVA/YUCA; PARSNIPS; TURNIPS

SUPERPOWERS: Nutrient-dense and satisfying. One of the few true comfort foods that's actually good for you, as long as you don't fry them.

SECRET WEAPONS: Calcium, iron, vitamins A, B, and C, selenium, beta carotene, magnesium, potassium, carotenoids, fiber.

POSERS: Candied sweet potatoes, french fries, hashbrowns, au gratin, loaded baked potato.

These root veggies are starchier and calorically dense in comparison to other vegetables, but they're also packed with antioxidants and fiber.

Potatoes

Even though they are white and get a bad rap, they are full of fiber, vitamins, and minerals and are so satisfying. But don't forget to eat the skin! You need that fiber!

MAKE THIS!

Baked fries! Just leave the skins on when prepping them to get the full potassium, fiber, and vitamin C.

Sweet Potatoes

Just one cup of baked sweet potatoes provides 400 percent of your daily vitamin A and half of your daily vitamin C intake, and while they taste sweet, they are totally okay on **Sugar Free 3**.

Corn

Depending on which expert you talk to, corn is considered both a starchy vegetable and a grain, which is why it's listed here, but you'll also see corn tortillas under whole grains. Whether you're eating it on the cob or air-popping it, it's great—filled with fiber and antioxidants. But when you grind it into corn flour or cornmeal, the calories start adding up quickly, so keep an eye on how much you're eating. And go organic if you're trying to avoid GMOs.

Winter Squash

True story: I am a pumpkin junkie—and not the pumpkin spice latte kind. In fact, I love all winter squash. When the leaves turn in autumn, I immediately crave kabocha or butternut squash soup. Squashes are also delicious roasted or in noodle form. The red-orange pigment in vegetables like squash and carrots comes from beta-carotene. Your body converts it to Vitamin A, to help with healthy skin and vision.

MAKE THIS!
Swap pasta out for butternut squash noodles!

Cassava/Yuca

Similar to a regular potato, yuca (or cassava) is another alternative. Also just as versatile as potatoes, these root veggies, often recognized by their long, cylindrical root shape, rough brown skin, and white flesh, are also filled with vitamin C.

What's the glycemic index (GI) and do I need to worry about it?

The glycemic index is a 1–100 scoring system that helps determine how quickly different carbohydrate-containing foods impact blood sugar. Glucose (sugar) rates 100. Meats and fats rate zero because they're carb-free. Anything below 55 is considered low GI. Anything above 70 is considered high GI.

While GI tells you how fast your blood sugar is affected, it doesn't tell you how high your blood sugar will go from a serving of food. To figure that out, scientists added a little math to the GI and created the glycemic load (GL). A score of 10 is a low GL; 20 or more is high.

If you find this all confusing, I can't say I disagree with you. That's why, with **SF3**, you don't have to worry about the GI or GL. Yes, some starchy carbs and fruits rank a little high on both scales, but that's part of the reason they're Allowed in Moderation instead of Totally Allowed. The lists are your guide.

Just focus on reducing added sugars and all those glycemic ratings should take care of themselves.

Whole Fruit

*BERRIES, APPLES, BANANAS, CHERRIES,
ORANGES, PEACHES; FREEZE-DRIED OR DEHYDRATED FRUIT
WITHOUT ADDED SUGARS*

SUPERPOWERS: Hydrating while satiating. Fruit is the natural way to satisfy your sweet tooth.

SECRET WEAPONS: Fiber, potassium, iron, antioxidants, vitamin C, hydration.

POSERS: Fruit juice, fruit juice concentrate, most fruit jams, dried fruit (with added sugar), fruit chews/candies.

The magic of fruit on **Sugar Free 3** is that within days of starting the program, you'll come to appreciate how sweet it really is. Green apples will taste like Jolly Ranchers. Tangerines will taste like orange gems. Be careful not to load up on too much fruit each day, particularly if weight loss is your goal. And I always recommend fresh over dried fruit. If you do eat dried fruit, keep in mind that getting rid of the water makes it more calorically dense, so eat less. Also, always read the label to check for added sugars!

A few of my go-tos are:

Berries. Fiber-packed, low in sugar, great raw, and perfect in oatmeal and shakes, they're just the best. Heat them up until they release their natural juice and then mix in with plain Greek yogurt.

Apples. Filled with fiber, I love them raw with a spoonful of nut butter or sprinkled with cinnamon or cardamom. Try our baked apple recipe on page 141.

Bananas. They're a tremendous source of potassium, and yummy too. Next time you buy a bunch, peel them and throw them in a resealable storage bag in the freezer. When you need a sweet treat, snap off half, let it thaw a minute, blend it—and prepare for guiltless custardy goodness. I also like to smear fresh slices with nut butter.

Cherries. Our test group participants loved this delicious fruit. Personal hack: I buy frozen cherries and snack on a few after dinner. Tastes like candy.

Unrefined Whole Grains

Brown Rice, Quinoa, Oats, Barley and other grains; Sprouted, Whole-Wheat, and Whole-Grain Breads, Pasta, Wraps, Corn Tortillas, and Crackers

SUPERPOWERS: Keeps the heart and bowel healthy.

SECRET WEAPONS: Protein, fiber, B vitamins, magnesium.

POSERS: Anything refined and enriched. Products that sound healthy but aren't, such as "multigrain," "7-grain," and "wheat"—if it doesn't have the word "whole" before it, it's probably refined!

Whole grains are the yin to the yang of beans. By themselves, they both provide plenty of nutrients, including fiber, but when combined, they form a complete protein, providing a balance of all nine essential amino acids similar to what you'll find in animal proteins. There's a reason that rice and beans are a staple combination in so many indigenous diets across the globe.

You don't need to eat them together with every meal, but getting both beans and grains at some point in your day is an excellent way to help meet your protein needs, especially if you don't eat a lot of meat, eggs, and dairy. Among the staples:

Brown Rice

The difference between brown and white rice perfectly illustrates the definition of a whole grain. Brown rice is literally the "whole" grain—bran, germ, endosperm and all, packed with belly-filling fiber and nutrients. White rice is rice with all that good stuff—aka the nutritious parts—removed. [*Insert sad trombone sound*] You're left with a carb that has very little nutritional value. Same goes for white pasta and white bread too. That's why brown rice is allowed on **Sugar Free 3**.

Quinoa

Ancient grains have waited thousands of years to suddenly be famous. Although technically a "pseudo grain," quinoa has been voted most popular. Gluten free, a fine source of protein, and easy to make, it's just one of the old-school grains now on shelves.

Oats

Packed with soluble fiber and good for your heart, oats or oatmeal are great high-fiber foods, old-fashioned or steel cut. But so many brands pack their flavored varieties with unnecessary sugars, you might as well be eating oatmeal cookies. Buy the plain varieties and sweeten with fruit.

Overnight Sensation *You know what's better than a recipe that takes just minutes to cook? A recipe that requires no cooking at all. That's why I adore overnight oats. Just combine some raw oats with a liquid, add some toppings, and pop in the fridge. By morning, instant breakfast or snack! Some of my favorite flavor combos are:*

▶ Oats, almond milk, peanut butter, chia seeds, and top with raspberries

▶ Oats, milk, blueberries, cinnamon, and top with shaved almonds

▶ Check out my scrumptious overnight oats recipe in Chapter 5.

Whole Grain Bread, Wraps, Pasta, and Crackers

It may surprise you to learn that most supermarket breads are made with sugar—yes, even the "multigrain," "enriched," or "healthy" varieties. Be sure to read labels carefully for two things: no added sugars and make sure it says "whole wheat" or "whole grain" not just "wheat" alone or "wheat flour." My top pick—for both the flavor and the fact that it's the easiest to find—is Ezekiel 4:9, made with whole wheat, barley, millet, lentils, soybeans, and spelt, all organic and sprouted. Sprouted grains are a great choice because the sprouting process unlocks many of the nutrients in a seed, making the resulting foods a nutritious option.

Note: You can get Ezekiel 4:9 in bread, pasta, wrap, English muffin, and cereal form.

Healthy Fats

Olive Oil and other Healthy Oils, NSA Mayonnaise, Avocado, Nuts and Seeds, Nut and Seed Butters

SUPERPOWERS: Keeps the heart healthy, controls appetite.

SECRET WEAPONS: Omega-3s, fiber, vitamins C, E, and K, magnesium, folate, B vitamins, monounsaturated fats.

POSERS: Nut butters with added sugar, oil, and salt, guacamole where avocado isn't the first ingredient, sweetened nuts, margarine.

It sounds like an oxymoron: "healthy fats." But that's just because food marketers have demonized the word "fat." In fact, we need fat to support cell structure, give our body energy, and help the body absorb nutrients.

Just keep in mind that fat is more calorically dense than other macronutrients. There are four calories in a gram of protein or carbohydrates while there are nine calories in a gram of fat. This doesn't make it unhealthy, it just means you can eat less of it to get all the nutrients you need out of it. Here are some of the healthiest.

Olive Oil

One of the pillars of the Mediterranean diet, olive oil is one of those foods that's super heart healthy while making everything it's added to delicious. If you're using it for salad dressings or dipping, use extra virgin. Extra-virgin olive oil is less processed and has the most nutrients. You can recognize it by its green tint. Unfortunately, those nutrients burn easily, so if you're cooking with olive oil, use the light variety.

Other Healthy Oils

With the exception of palm oil—which is high in a kind of saturated fat called palmitic acid—most vegetable-based oils are fine in moderation, but a few of my favorites include avocado oil, which is high in mono-unsaturated fats and is great for cooking; and walnut oil, which is high in polyunsaturated fats and great for adding flavor to salad dressings and pesto. GMOs play a big role in plant oils, so buy organic if that's a concern.

> *Cuckoo for Coconuts.* *Coconut is experiencing a renaissance lately. It seems like it's an ingredient in about half the things you find at the grocery store. Whether or not it's good for you is a matter of debate. The bulk of a coconut's calories come from fat. Specifically, it's a kind of saturated fat called lauric acid that some experts feel has positive health benefits while others feel is, well, just another saturated fat. Whether or not you use it, I will say that there are plenty of unsaturated fats out there—like you'll find in olive oil and avocados—that have more scientific evidence behind them pointing to how healthy they are.*

Avocado

Thanks to Instagram, the alligator-green superfood is superhot! And why not? It spreads well on toast, has no sodium or cholesterol, is loaded with monounsaturated fat and fiber, and contains nearly two dozen vitamins and minerals, including vitamins A and B6, potassium, copper, zinc, iron, magnesium, manganese, and phosphorous. Ripening and preserving an avocado can be tricky. Here are some tips to get the most use out of the finicky fruit:

◆ Need to ripen that avocado soon? Pop it in a paper bag. The fruit naturally produces ethylene gas, which gets trapped inside and speeds up the ripening process. You can also add in a kiwi or apple—both also produce ethylene—to speed things up.

◆ Split your avocado and need to store its other half? Not a problem. Spritz some lemon juice on the remaining half and store it in an airtight container. (Keeping the pit in doesn't really help except for the part that the pit physically covers.)

Nuts and Seeds

Sometimes you feel like a nut. And well you should, given how satisfying a handful of these "good fat" foods can be. Almonds, cashews, walnuts, pecans, pepitas (pumpkin seeds)—they may be high in calories, but they're so nutrient-rich it doesn't matter, as long as you practice a little moderation.

> **Go Green!** *My favorite nut, pistachios, seem to be everywhere, and they're one of the best nuts you can eat. One ounce of shelled nuts—about 49 kernels—is 159 calories, but that includes 7 grams of monounsaturated fat, 3 grams of fiber, 8 percent the daily value of potassium, and 25 percent the daily value of Vitamin B6.*

NUT AND SEED TIPS

▶ If you prefer them roasted, go with dry roasted.

▶ Try to buy unsalted or lightly salted.

▶ Don't go nuts with nuts as they are calorically dense.

▶ Steer clear of sugar-coated versions.

▶ Enjoy nut butter in a shake or on a fresh fruit or veggie.

Nut and Seed Butters

You'd think it'd be easy to navigate the grocery aisle when it comes to that simple childhood favorite, peanut butter. They're just mashed up peanuts, right? Nope. Read ingredient lists and you'll discover that nut and seed butters are Public Enemy Number One when it comes to added sugars and other garbage. When buying them, make sure they only contain nuts and/or seeds and maybe some salt.

Also keep in mind that nut and seed butters pack a big calorie punch. Eating even "one little spoonful more" can add hundreds of calories to your day, so less is more.

Dairy

YOGURT, CHEESE, COTTAGE CHEESE, MILK,
PLANT-BASED SUBSTITUTES

SUPERPOWERS: Some are high in protein, most promote bone health.

SECRET WEAPONS: Calcium, protein, probiotics, vitamin E, B12, magnesium.

POSERS: Anything with added sugars, including flavored yogurts, sweetened milk substitutes and, sadly, most chocolate milk.

For most people, the dairy we consume is as personal as the shoes we wear or our Netflix watch list. During **Sugar Free 3**, I've done my best to let you do you when it comes to these choices. (I'm talking about dairy. I couldn't care less about your television viewing habits.) Of course, you'll need to eliminate sugar-added choices like syrup-drenched "fruit" yogurt. Other than that, I try to buy organic .

Fat versus Fat Free? Fat is only half the issue here, so let's go there first. Over my years in the health magazine industry, I've seen full-fat dairy go from halo status to devil status back to halo status. The saturated fats in dairy are different from many other saturated fats, but the final verdict isn't in. On the other hand, everyone seems to consistently agree that the healthy, unsaturated fats you find in nuts, olive oil, and avocados are good stuff, so it's a much wiser bet making those your fats of interest.

The second half of the issue is the processing. Most low-fat and non-fat dairy is made by putting milk in a centrifuge and spinning the fat out. Reduced-fat and low-fat milk have some of the fat removed. Skim has all the fat removed. Unfortunately, many of the nutrients in milk are in the fat, so once it's removed, nutrients like vitamin A, vitamin D, and some of the proteins need to be added back in artificially. In other words, less fat means more processing.

Because vitamins like A, D, E, and K are fat-based, that also means that they are absorbed better into your body when consumed with a little fat. With this in mind, I recommend going low-fat or reduced-fat instead of skim.

And if you prefer full-fat, that's fine, but keep in mind that it's more caloric, so eat or drink less and make sure to balance it out with unsaturated fats.

I've broken dairy down into three sections to make things simple.

Low-Fat Plain Yogurt and Low-Fat or Reduced-Fat Cheeses

Recommendations: Low-fat Greek yogurt, low-fat cottage cheese, ricotta, feta, and mozzarella cheese.

Admittedly, these aren't really the kind of cheeses that you enjoy with a fine merlot—or that can make a pizza really sing. (Don't worry, full-fat Camembert and mozzarella come later.) The dairy listed here is less about indulgence and more about nutrition—albeit delicious nutrition.

Low-Fat Yogurt: Packed with probiotics to support a healthy gut, yogurt is also a solid source of calcium for bone health. Personally, I'm a fan of Greek yogurt, which differs from other yogurts because it goes through a straining process to remove the whey and reduces lactose, a natural sugar found in milk. This process also gives Greek yogurt its tartness and thickness. It's higher in protein than regular yogurt, but it also contains less calcium. Always be sure to get the "plain" variety and make sure there are no added sugars or artificial sweetener. Top it with some blueberries or raspberries and chia seeds. I also like to make a savory dip with it by sprinkling it with a spice mix called za'atar and drizzling olive oil over it.

Low-Fat or Reduced-Fat Cheese: Low-fat or reduced-fat cheeses are a good way to get your cheese fix without filling up on needless calories, and some of the newer brands taste *sooo* good. I personally can't tell the difference in taste between low-fat and full-fat ricotta and cottage cheese. They provide a complete protein, a hit of salt, and go great in recipes. (For example, you'll find fab reduced-fat feta cheeses that are great in salads.) Not to mention, for vegetarians, it's a solid alternative to meat proteins.

Vegan Yogurt and Cheese: For those living a vegan lifestyle, you'll find an array of new products made from almonds, cashews, soy, and coconut. Just make sure to look for plain varieties, and read the labels for hidden sugars and freakish ingredients you don't recognize.

Full-Fat Dairy

Recommendations: Any full-fat cheese you love and can't live without, whole milk, and ghee (clarified butter that's good for cooking).

Life is great, in part because of cheese. That's why it's allowed—but just enjoy it in moderation, like on your salad. I choose feta because I love it. It's lower in calories than Parmesan and other cheeses I dig, but as I will say throughout the book, the goal is for you to cut sugar and to complete the program, not feel tortured and deprived. If that means some cheese in your eggs or in your salad, go for it and enjoy it. You'll see some recipes with feta and goat cheese because I never want you to feel deprived—life is too short!

I also like to add a pat of grass-fed butter when cooking scrambled eggs or spread a bit on a nicely toasted slice of Ezekiel bread.

Milk (Cow and Plant-Based)

Recommendations: Low-fat milk; unsweetened plant-based milks.

I rarely recommend drinking your calories, so we've put milks under Allowed in Moderation with the hope you use it to add to your coffee or shake recipes. Lactose-free versions are also a great option since the natural milk sugar (lactose) has been broken down to help aid in digestion for those who are lactose intolerant. And every day there's a new type of plant or nut-based milk, so always be sure to read the ingredients list and opt for unsweetened versions.

Skim/Reduced/Low-Fat Milk: All three have their benefits. Skim has fewer calories, but it's the most processed. And the little bit of fat in reduced-fat or low-fat milk helps you better absorb fat-based vitamins in milk like vitamins A, D, E, and K. And note: While you'll see sugar grams on the label, there is no added sugar.

MILK BATTLE

Here's how the full fat-to-no-fat milks match up in terms of fat and calories per 8 fluid ounce serving.

Whole Milk (3.25%)

CALORIES: 149

FAT: 8 g

NATURAL SUGARS: 12 g

Low-Fat Milk (1%)

CALORIES: 102

FAT: 2 g

NATURAL SUGARS: 13 g

Reduced-Fat Milk (2%)

CALORIES: 122

FAT: 5 g

NATURAL SUGARS: 12 g

Skim (Fat-Free) Milk

CALORIES: 83

FAT: 0 g

NATURAL SUGARS: 12 g

Plant-Based Milks

In the dairy aisle you'll find a plethora of plant-based, non-dairy milk alternatives, perfect if you're lactose intolerant or vegan, including almond, oat, cashew, pea, coconut, and hemp, and all have some hefty benefits to boot. Here are some commonly used milk alternatives:

Unsweetened Almond Milk. The most popular non-dairy option out there, almond milk has less protein and calcium than cow's milk, but also has no cholesterol.

Unsweetened Oat Milk. Made from soaking oats in water, oat milk is a great alternative for those allergic to nuts. It's also a bit creamier, so it will give you a nicer consistency in that shake or cappuccino.

Unsweetened Soy Milk. Not as popular as it once was, but if you're looking for a non-dairy milk with a decent amount of protein, this is your best option. I also recommend buying organic, since that automatically means it's non-GMO.

Unsweetened Coconut Milk (in a carton, not a can). I'm talking about the coconut milk you find in a carton with all the other plant-based milk. Although it's mostly fat, it's diluted and fortified, so it's lower in calories and tends to be full of calcium and vitamins like B12 and A. On the other hand, the coconut milk or cream you'll find in a can, the type they put in piña coladas, is neither diluted nor fortified, so it's loaded with calories and fat and not the best choice.

Keep in mind that both kinds contain mostly saturated fat. As I mentioned above, some experts believe that coconut-based saturated fat is better for you than animal-based saturated fat, but it's up to you to make that choice.

TIPS

▶ Use alternative milks for coffee or your shakes only!

▶ Go organic if you want to avoid GMOs.

▶ Read labels and be sure no sugar has been added.

Coconut Water. You'd think coconut water would belong with juices, but it's a better option when doing **Sugar Free 3**. It's low in calories, high in electrolytes, and while it may contain natural sugar, it also contains fiber to help you absorb that sugar in a healthy way.

Other Flavor Enhancers

These flavor enhancers should be enjoyed in moderation because they have more calories and fat. And as always, be sure to read the ingredient list to make sure there are no added sugars.

Ketchup and Barbecue Sauce. Totally okay if you can find NSA versions, but be sure they haven't replaced the sugar with artificial sweeteners. But honestly, it's way easier to make your own. Be sure to check out our recipes, because who wants to live without these two.

Marinades. Enjoy your favorite flavors like Chinese, Japanese, Mediterranean, Indian, and more but make sure there's no sugar added.

Pasta Sauce. Not just for pasta anymore. No-sugar-added pasta sauces can add life to everything from grilled vegetables to quinoa to spiralized veggie "spaghettis." You may have to read a lot of labels to find one without sugar. Better still, check out our recipe on Openfit.

Salad Dressings. Beware of bottled varieties. Not only are most packed with sodium, but they're often made with honey or high fructose corn syrup. Instead, I whip up my own dressing with one part vinegar, one part extra virgin olive oil, a dash of lemon juice, salt, and pepper. For more options, check out our recipes on Openfit.

Stevia and Monk Fruit

STEVIA POWDER (LIQUID OR GREEN PACKETS)
MONK FRUIT (LIQUID OR PACKETS)

SUPERPOWERS: Provides sweetness—without a blood sugar spike.

SECRET WEAPONS: Zero calories.

POSERS: All artificial sweeteners.

"Michele," you're saying, "why are stevia and monk fruit allowed?" We debated allowing stevia and monk fruit, but here's why I allowed it. Unlike other chemical-laden sweeteners, these two come from natural sources. Stevia is a leaf, and monk fruit is, you guessed it, fruit. Therefore, I've allowed them on this plan.

Stevia—made from the *Stevia rebaudiana* plant—is 200 to 350 times sweeter than table sugar, and has been used to sweeten tea in South America for over 1,500 years.

What I love about monk fruit is that is contains zero sugars and yet its extract is 300 times sweeter. It's native to Asia and has been used in traditional Chinese medicine for generations.

Personally I can't drink coffee unless it's sweetened—I've tried. So I put a little stevia (my preferred brand is Sweet Leaf) in mine.

On **Sugar Free 3** you can use stevia or monk fruit for coffee or tea. Also note that you'll find NSA protein powders under Totally Allowed—including those sweetened with stevia and monk fruit—since they can play an important dietary role if you're active, on-the-go, or seeking more plant-based protein. You'll also find a few desserts, shakes, and Greek yogurt recipes to enjoy when you're craving something sweet.

Some stevia products are cut with junk. But these get a thumbs-up:

- *Sweet Leaf*
- *Trader Joe's*
- *365*
- *Whole Earth*

Smoothie Move. I recommend filling your diet with whole foods, but if you're in a rush, there's something to be said for whipping up a protein shake with your favorite unsweetened or Stevia-sweetened protein powder, such as the Openfit Plant-Based Protein Shake. I like to add greens and a healthy fat.

BARELY ALLOWED

These foods are tasty and technically free from added sugars, but they aren't the healthiest options—often packed with calories and unhealthy fats. They are sanctioned on this plan, but we recommend limiting to 1–2 servings per day—max.

High-Fat Proteins

FATTY CUTS OF GROUND BEEF, <85% LEAN PORK, LAMB, PORK SAUSAGE, BACON, <85% FAT GROUND BEEF, HOT DOGS, SALAMI, ETC.

We don't recommend these foods per se, but this is **Sugar Free 3**, not "Saturated Fat and Additive Free 3," so we're not going to ban these things. Just remember to keep them to a minimum, because they're not doing you any favors.

Here's a list of some of the fattiest cuts of beef, pork, and lamb.

- ◆ *Beef:* T-bone steak, rib-eye steak, rib roast, prime rib, short ribs, back ribs

- ◆ *Pork:* pork belly/bacon, back ribs, spareribs, pork shoulder

- ◆ *Lamb:* rack of lamb, lamb breast (aka belly), lamb neck, lamb shank

Deep-Fried and Other "Bad Fat" Foods
FRENCH FRIES, POTATO CHIPS, TORTILLA CHIPS, ADDITIVE-PACKED BOTTLED FAT-BASED DRESSINGS, PALM OIL

Honestly, all these foods get through on a technicality. Potato chips and french fries may be vegetables with no added sugars , but they are nutrient-poor and high in fat and calories. Same with tortilla chips and other fried foods that are hard to control, so please consume sparingly.

When it comes to bottled dressings, if they contain a giant list of mysterious ingredients, they're not doing you any good. Either look for ingredients you recognize or make your own. It's easier than you think.

As for palm oil, it's filled with a nasty saturated fat called palmitic acid. You'll also find this stuff in dairy and meat, but those have other benefits, whereas palm oil is easy to replace with something healthier.

NOT ALLOWED (for 3 weeks)

By now you realize all the foods you can eat and, as you can see, you will have plenty to eat.

The list below constitutes the Not Allowed Foods (aka everything you can't eat). There's a rhyme and reason to everything on this list. As you know by now, we're cutting added sugar, refined carbs, and artificial sweeteners. This is a great opportunity to get educated on what you're cutting and why. Once you have the knowledge, it will be easier to steer clear of these foods, hopefully beyond 21 days. To tell you the truth, after three weeks on the plan, I didn't miss them at all, well, maybe just my wine.

ADDED SUGARS

◆ *White Sugar, Brown Sugar, Honey, Agave or Maple Syrup, High Fructose Corn Syrup.* It's not just the white sugar you have to look out for. Whether it's brown sugar or says light, brown, or organic, your body breaks it down just like sugar. When you start reading labels you'll want to look for added sugar and its secret identities. For a complete list look at the sugar aka list on page 42.

◆ *Candy, Gum, and Chocolate (even dark chocolate).* These very sweet products are a no-brainer.

◆ *Pastries, Cookies, Cakes, Brownies, Muffins, Donuts (all the usual sugary baked goods).* Not only do they contain sugar, they also contain refined flour.

◆ *Sugar-Sweetened Condiments like Ketchup, Barbecue Sauce, and Most Salad Dressings, and Store-Bought Pasta Sauces.* While they may not taste or sound so sweet, many of your daily condiments contain sugar, high fructose corn syrup, or molasses and are not approved. Good news is we've created a **Sugar Free 3**-approved marinara, ketchup, barbecue sauce, and salad dressings. Check out Chapter 5.

◆ *Sweetened and Flavored Yogurts.* Whether vanilla, strawberry, or peach flavor, that "fruit on the bottom" is basically jam, which means sugar has been added.

◆ *Ice Cream, Frozen Yogurt, Sorbet, and Gelato.* Yummy and delicious, but sorry, they contain sugar. And be on the lookout for the light versions or high-protein versions, which have cane sugar or artificial sweeteners.

◆ *Dried Fruit with Added Sugar.* You may love Craisins but this dried fruit and many other dried fruits like mango and bananas contain added sugar, so be sure to read the labels. There are some varieties that have no added sugar.

◆ *Sugar-Sweetened Beverages, including Soda, Fruit Juice, Fruit Juice Concentrate, Sweet Tea, Lemonade, Sports Drinks, Sweetened Seltzers, Coffee Drinks, Store-Bought Smoothies, and Kombucha.* Soda has added sugar, fruit juice has been stripped of its fiber—I think you get the gist. Be sure to read the labels; even healthy drinks like kombucha have added sugar.

REFINED CARBS

Once you refine a grain—strip off the germ and bran—all you have left is the endosperm, which is mostly carbs but no fiber, so it behaves in your system much like sugar. Technically, white bread, bagels, wraps, and white pasta are made from "wheat," meaning they have been stripped of their fiber and nutrients. That's why it's Not Allowed. Look for the words "whole grain" and "whole wheat" when reading labels on bread, pasta, wraps, and crackers. If you see the word "wheat" alone on a label without the word "whole" before it, put it back.

I found a bag of popular pita chips that listed "organic wheat flour" as the main ingredient—sounds healthy, right? But it's a common trick for manufacturers to hope consumers confuse "wheat" for "whole wheat" or "organic" for healthful.

You'll also see breads that say "whole wheat" or sprouted breads that have sugar or high fructose corn syrup or honey added as well.

- ◆ **White Rice.** Wheat is wheat like corn is corn or rice is rice—it's just how it's processed that counts, which is why you can have brown rice, not white rice.

- ◆ **White Flour Products including Bread, Bagels, Pasta, Pita, Crackers, Pretzels, Most Cereals, and Pancake Batter.**
  - • If you're overwhelmed by label reading, a safe bet is Food for Life Ezekial Sprouted bread, which contains no added sugar.
  - • Be sure to check out my chapter and video about reading labels at Openfit.com/**SF3**.

- ◆ **Deep-Fried, Breaded, and Battered Foods like Chicken Parmesan, Tempura, Onion Rings, and Battered Fish.** If the deep-fried, unhealthy fats weren't enough reason to avoid them, these products are breaded with refined flour, so no thank you!

- ◆ **All Alcohol, including Wine and Beer. #SorryNotSorry!** Simply put, as far as your body is concerned, alcohol behaves similarly to a sugar or a refined carb—it's just empty calories. And your body will use it as an energy source rather than burning fat. Plus, people tend to make bad choices when they drink. And I want you to be in the strongest, most clear-minded position to make the best choices for the next three weeks!

ARTIFICIAL SWEETENERS

◆ *Artificial Sweeteners.* There are dozens of artificial or non-nutritive sweeteners out there, so if it promises to be sweet yet "sugar-free," "diet," "zero calorie," or "light," be careful. Some of the better known artificial sweeteners are sucralose (which you'll find in those yellow packs), aspartame and acesulfame potassium (both of which you'll find in blue packs), and saccharin (which you'll find in pink packs). We also include sugar alcohols in this group, so look out for ingredients ending with "itol."
Stevia and monk fruit are allowed.

◆ *Diet Soda, Seltzer, and Zero-Calorie Diet Drinks; Sugar-Free Diet Products like Yogurt, Sugar-Free Candy, Sugar-Free Gum and Mints.* Diet soda and many flavored seltzers and products like Crystal Light may tout zero calories but contain artificial sweeteners, so they're a no-go. Diet products like yogurt and other "sugar-free" products often contain artificial sweeteners; same goes for sugar-free gum and mints.

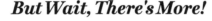

{ ***But Wait, There's More!***
For an extended list of
ALLOWED and NOT ALLOWED FOODS,
see the Appendix, page 218. }

FAQs

Answers to the Most Common Queries That Pop Up When on This Plan

Why no alcohol on the program—even tequila?

Let's get the obvious ones out of the way. Sugary cocktails, most beers, and sweeter wines all either contain sugar or the fiberless carbs that I've already explained behave like sugars.

That leaves us with hard alcohol, dry wine, and light beers. These three have little or no carbs or sugar to speak of, but they're still problematic for several reasons. First off, alcohol functions as a macronutrient, meaning the body uses it for energy as it does with protein, carbohydrates, and fat. There are seven calories per gram of alcohol. Fat has nine calories per gram. Carbs and protein have four calories per gram each. In this way, it behaves like fat. However, it also behaves like a carb because the body prefers using it for energy over fat. In this sense, it gets in the way of fat burning. So alcohol isn't closely related to sugar, but it shares some of its less admirable traits.

Second, alcohol is poison. The liver detoxifies it so it can be used as energy, but that process taxes the body. You're already giving your body a challenge by quitting sugar. Do you really need to add another challenge?

Finally, people tend to make bad choices when they drink. I want to set you up to make all the right, sugar-free choices for the next three weeks! Believe me, this sacrifice is no easy feat for me either.

Which form of alcohol is the best for my Mindful Indulgences?

Congratulations! You found the drinking loophole in **SF3**. Honestly, the best one is the one you'll enjoy the most. For most people, one alcoholic drink a week will do no harm, so drink what you like.

But if you seriously are looking for the "healthiest," your best bet is dry red wine. Yes, the alcohol is still there, but the sugar and other carbs aren't. Also, you get a little resveratrol and some polyphenols—phytonutrients shown to have various health benefits.

Soda's not allowed—I get that. But can I drink flavored club soda or seltzers?

The flavored sparkling water market is booming and they are healthier alternatives to soda. Unfortunately, not all are allowed on **Sugar Free 3**. Here's what's what:

- ◆ *Allowed:* Plain club soda; plain seltzer; seltzer enhanced with "natural essence" that has no sugar or calories on the label; flavor your seltzer yourself with a spritz of citrus.

- ◆ *Not Allowed:* Seltzer flavored with sugar; fruit juice (I know it's natural but it's still added sugar—minus the fiber you get from whole fruit); spiked (alcoholic) seltzers or those with artificial sweeteners.

- ◆ *Brands I love:* Poland Spring, Perrier, and Polar makes great seasonal flavors too!

Can I eat bread, pasta, wraps, and flour products?

Bread, pasta, and flour products are allowed if you know what to look for.

This isn't a no-carb or low-carb plan. With this in mind, if it's a good, fibrous carb, I see no reason to exclude it. Unless you have some sort of gluten issue, whole grain bread and other whole grain products can be a yummy, nutritious part of anyone's diet.

Here's the scoop: If you see the word "wheat" alone on a label without the word "whole" before it, walk away. And by the same token, if you see "whole wheat" or "whole grain" on a label, be sure to make sure there is no sugar (in any form) on the ingredient list. Marketing "organic wheat flour" as the main ingredient is a common trick used to confuse us.

You'll also see whole wheat or sprouted grain products that have sugar or high fructose corn syrup or honey added in as well.

One safe bet is Ezekial sprouted bread, which contains no added sugar. *Be sure to check out my video at Openfit.com/**SF3**.*

Seriously, I can have popcorn and corn tortilla chips?

Technically, yes, because these are made of whole grains and generally don't contain added sugars, refined grains, or artificial sweeteners. But frankly, tortilla chips and their tuberous cousins—potato chips—aren't good for you at all. So eat if you must, but opting for some air-popped popcorn is a better choice.

Why is brown rice okay?

The reason is, like whole wheat, it retains the fiber, and therefore acts less like a sugar than white rice, in which the fiber is stripped away.

Are starches allowed?

Yes. This question came up in every test group. You'll notice it on so many food products when you start reading labels, especially items like wraps and crusts. Starches like potato starch and corn starch are used in food products and recipes as a thickener or a stabilizer. Starch is technically a complex carbohydrate, not a sugar. And while I wouldn't really classify it as a health food, it's not used in problematic levels and it's not a sweetener, so I let it go. Same with pectin.

Mayonnaise under Healthy Fats? Really?

True mayonnaise consists of three things: egg yolks, oil, and something acidic like lemon juice or vinegar to help it emulsify. Technically, all these things are on the Allowed in Moderation list, so that's where mayo should live. The only problem is that store-bought mayonnaise tends to have an ingredient list far beyond these three items—and the extra stuff is rarely good for you, including added sugars. So read the label. If it contains eggs, a healthy oil, vinegar or lemon juice, and maybe a few other things you recognize and trust, please enjoy it in moderation. If it's filled with additives, consider it Barely Allowed. And if it contains added sugars, put it back.

Why can't I have alcohol, but red and white wine vinegar are allowed?

I'm a big fan of salads and hence vinegar. Although vinegar is made from alcohol, during the fermentation process most of that alcohol is converted to acetic acid and water. Only a trace amount remains— certainly not enough to cause any issues. So rejoice! Almost all vinegar is allowed, like white, white wine, champagne, red wine, and apple cider. The only vinegar to look out for is balsamic, because it contains grape must, which behaves like added sugar.

Is eating too much whole fruit bad? Isn't it full of sugar?

Fruit is better than any refined sugar because it's a whole food that also comes with fiber, vitamins, minerals, and antioxidants. Still, you don't want to overconsume it. An apple a day keeps the doctor away but an apple, a banana, 40 grapes, 20 strawberries, and a kiwi is overkill.

Why is fresh or frozen fruit allowed, but fruit juice and juice concentrate aren't?

The alchemy of fruit is amazing—a perfect balance of sugar, fiber, water, and other nutrients. When you start messing with that balance, things go downhill fast. With fruit juice, the fiber is gone, so the sugars hit your bloodstream unregulated. Juice concentrate intensifies the problem by decreasing the water, which decreases the volume, meaning you can consume more sugar calories in less food. Bad news.

Do I have to pay attention to serving size?

The good news about this program is there is no calorie counting or portion control required, but that does not mean you can eat unlimited amounts of any food. Below are a few examples to use as guidelines. In general, eat until satisfied, but keep these rules of thumb in mind, especially if you're trying to lose or maintain your weight:

- ◆ *Protein:* About the size of a deck of cards is a serving. Feel free to enjoy 1–2 servings at any given meal.

- ◆ *Fruit:* Start with 1 whole fruit or 1 cup of chopped fruit or berries.

- ◆ *Vegetables:* 1–3 cups of most veggies; 1 cup for starchy veggies or 1 medium potato.

- ◆ *Healthy Fat:* 1 tbsp of oil is a serving, 1 oz. of nuts, ¼ avocado.

Do I need to care about the glycemic index?

With **SF3**, you don't have to worry about the glycemic index—a ranking of carbohydrates in foods according to how they affect your blood glucose levels—or glycemic load. Yes, some starchy carbs and fruits rank a little high on both scales, but that's part of the reason they're Allowed in Moderation instead of Totally Allowed. The lists are your guide.

Just focus on reducing added sugars, and all those glycemic ratings should take care of themselves. For more information on the glycemic index, see page 78.

Some ingredients have weird names. Are these allowed?

◆ *Xantham gum?* Xantham gum is a plant-based additive used for thickening foods. It's a complex carb, not a sugar. It's fine on **SF3**.

◆ *Carrageenan?* Carrageenan is another plant-based thickener. It's made from seaweed. Again, not a sugar and okay on **SF3**.

◆ *Erythritol and Maltitol?* If you see an "itol" at the end of it, that means it's a sugar alcohol, which isn't a great name for them since they're neither sugar nor alcohol. They are, however, chemically processed artificial sweeteners, so they're a no-go.

◆ *Maltodextrin?* Maltodextrin is a food additive made from starch that's usually used as a thickener or as a preservative. It's not often used as a sweetener, but it does contain some sugar, so it's something to avoid during **SF3**.

Does having stevia or monk fruit trigger you to crave more sweets?

There's research showing artificial sweeteners trick the brain into thinking it's received carb calories, and once the brain realizes it didn't get those calories, it triggers cravings for them. This research doesn't determine whether natural non-caloric sweeteners, such as monk fruit and stevia, also cause this issue, but it's logical to assume they might.

So while stevia and monk fruit, both derived from plants, don't cause all the issues that sugar causes and they're generally considered safer than most artificial sweeteners, there's still a risk of triggering cravings when you use them, so be ready.

Can I do Sugar Free 3 and do intermittent fasting?

Sure. It's your call.

What do I do if I am hungry or craving something sweet?

Read Chapter 8!

Can I chew gum? Even if it's sugarless?

Sorry, no. Most gum is made with sugar or artificial sweeteners—and they're not **SF3** approved.

Eat This, Not That! On Sugar Free 3

A FEW GROCERY ITEMS consistently tripped up those who have done **Sugar Free 3**, so I asked my friend Dave Zinczenko and his team at Eat This, Not That! (eatthis.com) to put together this quick list to clear things right up.

Bread

▶ *Not That!:* Bread, by definition, is made from flour and water. Therefore, most breads are a no-go for three weeks; the majority of them are made from refined flour and often contain added sugars. That said, this plan isn't Carb Free 3. Bread is allowed in moderation! As long as you...

▶ *Eat This Instead:* ...enjoy an NSA bread made from whole or sprouted grains. Among the brands found in most major supermarkets, the one you're most likely to find is Food for Life brands like Ezekiel 4:9, made with wheat, barley, millet, lentils, and other sprouted grains. You'll mostly find it in a fridge case, not the bread aisle. (Why refrigerated? Because without artificial preservatives, it spoils faster.) You could also make your own bread; there's a recipe in the Openfit app.

Or get creative with what "bread" means. Amber H. from our test group made a cheeseburger between two roasted slices of sweet potato! Others have tried lettuce wraps, coconut wraps, and even portobello mushroom caps. It looked yummier than her husband's, made with white toast. Check out the sweet potato toast in Chapter 5.

Pre-Prepared Protein

▶ *Not That!:* This surprised a lot of **Sugar Free 3** shoppers—many pre-cooked proteins, like packages of chicken or turkey, have sugar added. This is often to "preserve freshness" or add flavor.

▶ *Eat This Instead:* Read the label carefully. Now you can find many options without added sugar or just buy your proteins straight up, not marinated or pre-made, using the guide in Chapter 5.

Plant-Based Milks

▶ *Not That!:* Many major alternative milks—almond, rice, soy, hemp, cashew, oat, coconut—are made with sugar (yes, not just the vanilla or chocolate flavors, but even the "plain" or "enriched" varieties, too!) It's often listed as organic evaporated cane syrup or cane sugar.

▶ *Eat This Instead:* It's simple. Buy the unsweetened version. Blend it into a fruit and protein powder shake if you need a hit of sweetness.

Ketchup

▶ *Not That!:* Ketchup without sugar is very hard to find. And most of the "sugar-free" varieties contain sucralose (an artificial sweetener) or balsamic vinegar, which itself contains sugar. Sneaky!

▶ *Eat This Instead:* Rather than scout the aisles looking for this elusive sugar-free sauce, you can improvise and add a dab of NSA pasta sauce to a turkey burger or use the NSA ketchup recipe developed for this program.

Soup

▶ *Not That!:* Did grandma put sugar into your chicken soup? Didn't think so. But some food companies load their chicken soup with not one, but two forms of sugar. You'll also find it in many tomato soups, meat-based soups and "creamy" soups.

▶ *Eat This Instead:* Instead of "home style," go homemade, if you have the time. (There's a belly-warming recipe at Openfit. com/**SF3**). Or buy a pre-made bone or veggie broth (fresh is better, but boxed will do) and use it as a base for your soup. Just add protein, veggies, herbs, and spices. Otherwise, check the label of canned soups and look for meats, veggies, herbs, spices, water, salt—and little else.

Bottled and Canned Beverages

▶ *Not That!:* Sugar water is big business because it's cheap to make and easy to sell. That's why you'll find it sold under many different names, many with a health halo. Many coffee and matcha tea drinks add sugar to reduce the bitterness. And most store-bought kombuchas are made with sugars like organic evaporated cane juice. And since fruit juice isn't allowed on **Sugar Free 3**, even naturally-sweetened waters are not allowed.

▶ *Drink This Instead:* Fresh tap, filtered, bottled, or sparkling water, unsweetened flavored seltzers, tea, and coffee are all you need to caffeinate and hydrate healthily.

Chocolate

▶ *Not That!:* "Hellllloooooo!!!! What kind of chocolate is allowed? #ItsAnEmergency" wrote April B. from a Trader Joe's. She'd taken a photo of the store's Belgian chocolates, milk chocolate caramel crunch medallions, and soft honey nougat with almonds. Needless to say, none of that is allowed on **Sugar Free 3**. Chocolate is traditionally made with sugar, so no traditional chocolates are allowed.

▶ *Eat This Instead:* If you really need your fix, indulge in Lily's (made with stevia), which we've seen at Whole Foods, or order some Choczero (made with monk fruit), available at online retailers. The new Openfit Plant-Based Protein Shake comes in chocolate. Or have a little dark chocolate as your Mindful Indulgence.

*For more brand name foods, visit the back of the book or Openfit.com/**SF3**.*

CHAPTER

5

RECIPES AND WHAT TO EAT

Three Delicious Meal Plans to Fit Your Lifestyle

T**HIS PLAN FITS** into any lifestyle. Not everyone has time at every feeding interval to whip up a meal (some days, I barely have time to eat one). That's why we created three ways to do the program, and on the pages that follow, a seven-day sample of each:

◆ *Like to Cook.* For those who love food and are interested and willing to experiment in the kitchen and cook. Use our recipes, all taking 30 minutes or less, or use your own favorites to create sugar-free meals.

♦ ***Willing to Cook.*** This is the semi-homemade route, which is even quicker and easier using pre-cut, pre-washed, and even pre-cooked food to make your meals

♦ ***Don't Cook.*** Good news! You don't have to cook on **Sugar Free 3**— order in, take out, or dine out with some suggestions, plus a full dining out chapter ahead.

With recipes as simple and yummy as the ones in this chapter, everyone from gourmet cooks to masters of the microwave will be stoked to get chopping. The list of things our recipe developers were able to dream up is impressive: energy-boosting breakfasts, never-boring lunches (no sad desk salads in sight!), delicious dinners, and scrumptious snacks—all without added sugars. But feel free to experiment with your own favorite recipes.

When you cook...

You'll be in charge of what's going into your food, because you're hand-selecting every ingredient and crafting it into something gratifying, unlike in restaurants, where sugar can be added. And you'll realize how novice-proof these recipes really are. For most, all you'll need is what you already have: an oven, a pan, or a toaster oven.

Either way, review all three plans and determine what works for you. You can also mix and match between the three based on your schedule. And this isn't even the half of it. Go to Openfit.com/**SF3** and you'll find dozens more exclusive recipes that take mere minutes to throw together, along with videos to guide you.

Still Hungry? Add 1–2 snacks a day like hard-boiled eggs, Greek yogurt and fruit, fruit and nut butter, veggies and hummus, or an Openfit Plant-Based Protein Shake!

LIKE TO COOK
7-Day Sample of Recipes You Can Make at Home

	BREAKFAST	LUNCH	DINNER
Monday	Sweet Potato Toast with "Crispy" Egg	Greek Chopped Salad with Shrimp	Lemon-Thyme Sheet Pan Roast Chicken with Shallots and Carrots
Tuesday	Eggs, Avocado, and Sautéed Greens (with optional Za'atar spice)	Chicken Caesar Salad with Pumpkin Seeds	Classic Beef Burger with Sweet Potato Fries
Wednesday	Coconut-Cashew Overnight Oats	Curried Cauli Rice with Roasted Veggies and Almonds	Grilled Chicken Paillard with Red Wine Vinaigrette over Arugula
Thursday	Almond Berry Parfait	Spiced Chicken Kebabs over Cauli-Rice-Tabouli	Grilled Flank Steak with Asparagus
Friday	Greek Egg Scramble	Juicy Turkey Burgers with Avocado and Turkey Bacon	Salmon with Herb Puree and Roasted Brussels Sprouts
Saturday	Speedy Shakshouka	Sesame Salmon with Fennel and Orange Salad	Egg Roll in a Bowl
Sunday	Pumpkin Ricotta Pancakes	BLT Sweet Potato Toast	Broiled Lemon Garlic Shrimp with Quinoa, Tomatoes, and Spinach

KISS (Keep It Simple, Silly)

I am super-busy but also like to eat healthfully, which is why I try to mostly eat the same things day to day to keep it simple. It just works. Whether that's eggs and greens most weekdays or Greek salad three days in a row until I get bored, it's simple to shop for, simple to prepare, and helps me stay consistent. So streamline your cooking and pick 1–2 breakfasts to enjoy each week, 1–2 lunches, and 1–2 dinners.

BREAKFAST

SWEET POTATO TOAST
with "Crispy" Egg
(Makes 1 serving)

◆Your favorite breakfast sandwich gets a healthy makeover when you serve it on sweet potato "toast" instead of bread. Slice a sweet potato lengthwise, then pop the slices in your toaster or toaster oven for an amazing sweet-savory alternative!

TOTAL TIME: **15 MINUTES** / PREP TIME: **5 MINUTES** / COOKING TIME: **10 MINUTES**

2 slices large sweet potato, ¼ inch thick
1 tsp. olive oil, divided
2 large eggs
Sea salt (or Himalayan salt) and ground black pepper (to taste; optional)
Cilantro or other fresh herbs (to taste; optional)
Pickled onions (optional)

1. Brush sweet potato slices lightly with ¼ tsp. olive oil and season with salt and pepper to taste (if desired).

2. Toast the sweet potato slices on the darkest toast setting in toaster or toaster oven and toast 2 or 3 times, flipping each time for even toasting, until slices are lightly browned and fork tender.

3. While sweet potato slices are toasting, heat the remaining olive oil in a small nonstick pan over high heat.

4. Add eggs; cook 4 to 5 minutes or to desired doneness.

5. Top each toasted sweet potato slice with 1 egg and herbs.

6. Top with pickled onions: (2 Tbsp. minced red onion with 1 tsp. white wine vinegar). Toss together onion with vinegar in a small bowl. Set aside.

TIPS: *OPTIONAL ADD-ONS*

▶ Top with shredded cheese or hot sauce, if desired

▶ Plain Sweet Potato Toast is also delicious topped simply with nut butter to satisfy your sweet tooth at breakfast.

▶ Sweet Potato Toast can be prepped ahead of time and reheated in the toaster.

BREAKFAST

EGGS, AVOCADO & SAUTÉED GREENS
(with optional Za'atar spice)
(Makes 1 serving)

◆ Give your basic eggs and greens an amazing flavor boost with a sprinkle of za'atar. This Middle Eastern seasoning features a flavorful mix of dried herbs, spices, and sesame seeds and is also delicious on hummus, roasted veggies, or grilled chicken or fish.

TOTAL TIME: **11 MINUTES** / PREP TIME: **3 MINUTES** / COOKING TIME: **8 MINUTES**

Olive oil cooking spray
4 cups baby spinach or baby kale
2 large eggs, whisked
¼ avocado, sliced
½ tsp za'atar, optional as desired

1. Coat a small nonstick sauté pan with olive oil cooking spray and heat over high heat.

2. Add spinach or kale and cook, stirring frequently, for 2–3 minutes or until wilted. Remove to a bowl and set aside.

3. Reduce heat to low and coat pan with additional cooking spray.

4. Add eggs and cook, whisking frequently, for 3–5 minutes or until fluffy and cooked through.

5. Serve eggs and greens topped with avocado, seasoned with salt and pepper to taste, and sprinkled with za'atar.

TIP
▶ Za'atar can be found at most upscale supermarkets or online too.

BREAKFAST

COCONUT-CASHEW OVERNIGHT OATS
(Makes 1 serving)

 Vegan

◆ Prep some overnight oats before bed for a speedy grab-and-go breakfast in the morning! Luscious cashew butter and crunchy cacao nibs combine deliciously to satisfy your sweet cravings.

TOTAL TIME: **OVERNIGHT TO REST** / PREP TIME: **5 MINUTES** / COOKING TIME: **1 MINUTE**

½ cup old-fashioned oats

⅔ cup unsweetened vanilla coconut milk

¼ tsp. cinnamon, additional for garnish

Pinch salt

1 Tbsp. cashew butter

1 Tbsp. cacao nibs (optional)

1. Combine oats, coconut milk, cinnamon, and salt in a small container. Cover and refrigerate overnight.

2. Microwave cashew butter for 1 minute in a small bowl and drizzle over oats.

3. Top with cacao nibs (if you like) and enjoy.

TIPS

▶ You can enjoy overnight oats chilled, at room temperature, or warmed up for a few minutes in the microwave for a hot breakfast alternative.

▶ Experiment and jazz up your oats with different nuts and spices and even fruit.

▶ If you don't like coconut milk, you can replace with unsweetened almond milk.

BREAKFAST

ALMOND BERRY PARFAIT

(Makes 1 serving)

◆ Treat yourself to a gorgeous dessert-like breakfast! Greek yogurt is layered with juicy mixed berries, drizzled with almond butter, and topped with crunchy toasted almonds in this make-ahead meal.

TOTAL TIME: **10 MINUTES** / PREP TIME: **10 MINUTES** / COOKING TIME: **1 MINUTES**

1 cup Greek yogurt (plain, 2%)

1 cup mixed berries

1 Tbsp. almond butter

1 Tbsp. sliced almonds, toasted

1. Layer ⅓ cup yogurt and ⅓ cup berries in a glass or bowl. Repeat to make 3 layers.

2. Microwave almond butter in a small glass bowl for 1 minute to thin.

3. Drizzle almond butter over top of berries, top with toasted almonds and enjoy.

TIPS

▶ Feel free to use NSA non-dairy yogurt, such as coconut.

▶ This parfait would also be delicious with diced peaches, kiwi, or mango instead of the berries—or any fruit, really!

▶ Toast sliced almonds ahead of time and store in a jar in your fridge.

BREAKFAST

GREEK EGG SCRAMBLE
(Makes 1 serving)

◆ This simple but flavorful one-pan scramble will be your go-to on busy mornings! Try a mix of colored grape tomatoes for an eye-pleasing look.

TOTAL TIME: **12 MINUTES** / PREP TIME: **5 MINUTES** / COOKING TIME: **7 MINUTES**

1 tsp. olive oil, divided (or cooking spray)

1 small shallot, sliced

4 cups baby spinach

3 large eggs, beaten

2 Tbsp. crumbled feta cheese

1 cup grape or cherry tomatoes, halved

1 Tbsp. chopped fresh oregano (or 1 tsp. dried)

1. Heat ½ tsp. olive oil in a medium nonstick sauté pan on medium-high heat.

2. Add shallot and baby spinach and cook for 2–3 minutes or until spinach wilts. Remove to a bowl and set aside.

3. Add remaining ½ tsp. olive oil to pan and reduce heat to low.

4. Add eggs and cook, whisking constantly, for 2–3 minutes or until cooked through and fluffy.

5. Stir in feta, reserved spinach mixture, grape tomatoes, and oregano.

6. Season to taste with salt and pepper (if desired) and enjoy.

TIPS

▶ Swap in any mix of greens or veggies you have on hand for this such as kale, chard, or arugula.

▶ You can also use goat cheese in place of feta and other herbs such as chopped basil, cilantro, dill, tarragon, parsley, or chives.

BREAKFAST

SPEEDY SHAKSHOUKA
(Makes 1 serving)

◆ Shakshouka (or shakshuka) is Middle Eastern slang for "stew"—usually served as we do here with slow-simmered eggs on top. This hearty one pan makes for a satisfying savory breakfast or brunch.

TOTAL TIME: **24 MINUTES** / PREP TIME: **5 MINUTES** / COOKING TIME: **19 MINUTES**

1 tsp. olive oil
¼ cup diced onion
¼ cup diced red pepper
1 tsp. cumin
½ tsp. smoked paprika
1½ cup canned diced fire-roasted tomatoes
2 cups baby spinach
2 large eggs
2 Tbsp. crumbled goat cheese
Cilantro or parsley for garnish (optional)

1. Heat olive oil over medium heat in a small non-stick sauté pan.
2. Add onion, pepper, cumin, and smoked paprika.
3. Season with salt and pepper (if desired) and sauté for 5–7 minutes, stirring often, until soft.
4. Add tomatoes and spinach and stir to combine.
5. Cook for 2 minutes to wilt spinach and bring mixture to a simmer.
6. Crack eggs into tomato mixture, cover pan, and continue to simmer for 5-10 minutes or until whites are set.
7. Top with goat cheese, season with additional salt and pepper (if desired), and garnish with optional herbs.

TIP
▶ If you don't like the smoky flavor, skip the fire-roasted tomatoes and swap in plain canned diced tomatoes instead.

BREAKFAST

PUMPKIN RICOTTA PANCAKES

(Makes 1 serving)

◆ Enjoy all the flavor of your favorite pumpkin pie for breakfast! These super-moist and delicate pancakes are perfect for a cozy weekend brunch.

TOTAL TIME: **15 MINUTES** / PREP TIME: **5 MINUTES** / COOKING TIME: **10 MINUTES**

⅓ cup pumpkin puree

¼ cup part skim ricotta

1 large egg

¼ tsp. pumpkin pie spice

¼ tsp. cinnamon

¼ tsp. baking powder

Stevia or monk fruit, optional to taste, in batter if desired

1 Tbsp. toasted chopped pecans

1. Whisk together pumpkin puree, ricotta, egg, pumpkin pie spice, cinnamon, baking powder, and optional sweetener in a small bowl.

2. Coat a large nonstick skillet with cooking spray and set over medium heat.

3. Pour batter into pan to make 4 small pancakes.

4. Cook for 4–5 minutes per side, gently flipping when bubbles form in the center of each pancake.

5. Serve dusted with additional cinnamon or pumpkin pie spice and topped with pecans.

TIP

▶ Serve with banana, toasted walnuts, or a dollop of NSA yogurt.

LUNCH

GREEK CHOPPED SALAD
with Shrimp
(Makes 1 serving)

◆ This easy recipe combines all the flavors of your favorite Greek salad in a colorful crunchy bowl. You can skip the shrimp to make this vegetarian.

TOTAL TIME: **10 MINUTES** / PREP TIME: **10 MINUTES** / COOKING TIME: **0 MINUTES**

1 cup chopped romaine lettuce

½ cup chopped red peppers

½ cup chopped cucumber

½ cup halved grape tomatoes

5 oz. poached or grilled shrimp

2 Tbsp. minced red onion

1 Tbsp. crumbled feta cheese

Chopped fresh mint or oregano (optional)

Greek Vinaigrette

1 tsp. red wine vinegar

2 tsp. olive oil

1 tsp. dijon mustard

1. Toss together romaine lettuce, peppers, cucumber, and tomatoes in a salad bowl.

2. Whisk together Greek Vinaigrette ingredients and drizzle over the top.

3. Season to taste with salt and pepper (if desired).

4. Top salad with shrimp, onion, crumbled feta cheese, and optional fresh mint or oregano.

TIPS

▶ Pick up Persian or Kirby cucumbers at the supermarket to have just the right amount to dice.

▶ If you're not a shrimp fan, just swap in cubed cooked chicken breast instead.

LUNCH

CHICKEN CAESAR SALAD
with Pumpkin Seeds
(Makes 1 serving)

◆ You won't believe how rich and luscious this light yogurt-based caesar dressing is! Just add your favorite greens and some grilled chicken for a speedy, super yummy lunch. Toasted pumpkin seeds add crunch in lieu of the typical croutons.

TOTAL TIME: **5 MINUTES** / PREP TIME: **5 MINUTES** / COOKING TIME: **0 MINUTES**

For Dressing:
- 2 Tbsp. Greek yogurt (plain, 2%)
- 2 tsp. olive oil
- 1 tsp. lemon juice
- 3 Tbsp. fresh grated parmesan, divided
- ½ tsp. minced garlic
- ½ tsp. anchovy paste (optional)

For Salad:
- 2½ cups chopped romaine lettuce or baby kale
- 6 oz. grilled chicken breast, sliced
- 1 Tbsp. toasted pumpkin seeds

1. Whisk together all dressing ingredients, reserving 1 Tbsp. parmesan for garnish.
2. Pour dressing over greens, toss to coat, and season to taste with salt and pepper (if desired).
3. Top salad with chicken, pumpkin seeds, and reserved 1 Tbsp. parmesan.

TIPS
▶ Imported aged Parmesan Reggiano will give this dish the best flavor, or skip if you prefer.

▶ Pick up grilled chicken at your local market or try our simple chicken marinade to prep your own grilled chicken ahead of time.

LUNCH

VEGAN CURRIED CAULI RICE
with Roasted Veggies & Almonds
(Makes 1 serving)

 Vegan

◆ A mix of tender roasted broccoli, mushroom, and carrot compliments crunchy, lightly spiced cauliflower rice in this easy vegan dinner.

TOTAL TIME: **15 MINUTES** / PREP TIME: **5 MINUTES** / COOKING TIME: **10 MINUTES**

1 cup small broccoli florets

1 cup ¼"-thick sliced carrots

1 cup chopped button mushrooms

1 small shallot, cut into wedges

2 tsp. curry powder, divided

¾ cup cauliflower rice

2 tsp. coconut oil, melted, divided

½ tsp. lime juice

1 Tbsp. toasted sliced almonds

Lime wedge and cilantro for garnish (if desired)

1. Preheat oven or toaster oven to 450 degrees.

2. Toss together broccoli, carrots, mushrooms, and shallot on a small baking pan lined with parchment.

3. Sprinkle with 1 tsp. curry powder and spray with cooking spray. Season as desired with salt and pepper.

4. Roast for 10 minutes or until browned.

5. Combine cauliflower rice, remaining ½ tsp curry powder, 1 tsp. coconut oil, and lime juice in a small bowl.

6. Top curried cauli rice with roasted vegetables.

7. Drizzle with remaining 1 tsp. coconut oil and top with toasted almonds and optional lime wedge and cilantro.

TIPS

▶ Feel free to sub your favorite veggies.

▶ Add a delicious protein for a more filling meal.

LUNCH

SPICED CHICKEN KEBABS
over Cauli-Rice Salad
(Makes 1 serving)

◆ Juicy chicken kebabs are paired with a crunchy "tabouli-style" salad using pre-made fresh cauliflower rice. Don't skip the fresh herbs in this recipe—they make it a standout!

TOTAL TIME: **15 MINUTES** / PREP TIME: **10 MINUTES** / COOKING TIME: **10 MINUTES**

4 oz. chicken breast, cut into 1½" cubes

1¼ tsp. cumin, divided

1¼ tsp. coriander, divided

1 cup fresh cauliflower rice

½ cup halved grape tomatoes

½ cup diced cucumber

¼ cup chopped parsley or mint

3 Tbsp. minced red onion or shallot

2 tsp. olive oil

2 tsp. lemon juice

1. Skewer chicken breast cubes onto 2 small or 1 large skewer.

2. Sprinkle chicken with ¼ tsp. cumin, ¼ tsp. coriander, and salt and pepper (if desired).

3. Heat a grill pan over high heat and coat with cooking spray.

4. Grill chicken for 3–4 minutes per side or until cooked through.

5. Toss together cauliflower rice, tomatoes, cucumber, parsley or mint, onion, olive oil, lemon juice, and remaining 1 tsp. cumin and 1 tsp. coriander, and season with salt and pepper (if desired).

TIPS

▶ If you can't find pre-made cauliflower rice (usually in the freezer section), it's easy to DIY. Just pulse cauliflower florets in a food processor or grate a whole head of cauliflower on a box grater.

▶ If need be, sub in quinoa for the cauli-rice.

LUNCH

JUICY TURKEY BURGERS
with Avocado & Turkey Bacon
(Makes 1 serving)

◆ Give basic lean ground turkey burgers an amazing flavor boost with these quick mix-ins and enjoy the incredible results.

TOTAL TIME: **15 MINUTES** / PREP TIME: **5 MINUTES** / COOKING TIME: **10 MINUTES**

---

4 oz. raw ground 93% lean turkey

¼ cup minced mushrooms

1 Tbsp. minced shallot or onion

1 slice turkey bacon

¼ avocado, sliced

Lettuce leaves and tomato for serving (optional)

1. Combine ground turkey, mushrooms, and shallot and form into a patty. Season to taste with salt and pepper (if desired).

2. Coat a grill pan or sauté pan with cooking spray and cook burger over medium-high heat for 4–5 minutes per side, or until no longer pink inside.

3. Cook bacon for 2–3 minutes alongside burger (or microwave on a paper towel–lined plate for 2 minutes or until crispy).

4. Serve burger on lettuce leaves and tomato topped with bacon and avocado.

TIPS

▶ Try adding minced fresh herbs to your turkey burger for even more flavor.

▶ Be sure to cook bacon and drain fat.

▶ Have fun with toppings for your burger like quick pickled onions, our **SF3** ketchup, mustard, pickles, or hot sauce.

LUNCH

SESAME SALMON
with Fennel & Orange Salad
(Makes 1 serving)

◆ Juicy oranges pair perfectly with crunchy fennel and an Asian-inspired vinaigrette in this filling lunch salad. Simple roasted salmon makes the perfect protein topper.

TOTAL TIME: **5 MINUTES** / PREP TIME: **5 MINUTES** / COOKING TIME: **0 MINUTES**

---

1 cup baby spinach

½ cup thinly sliced fennel

1 navel orange, peeled and sliced

6 oz. roasted salmon filet

1 tsp. toasted sesame seeds

Sesame Vinaigrette

2 tsp. NSA rice wine vinegar

2 tsp. sesame oil

½ tsp. minced ginger

1 chopped scallion, divided

1. Combine spinach, fennel, and orange slices in a salad bowl.

2. Whisk together Sesame Vinaigrette ingredients (reserving scallion greens) and drizzle over salad. Season to taste with salt and pepper.

3. Top with pre-roasted salmon, scallion greens, and sesame seeds.

TIP

▶ If you're packing this the night before for work, put the dressing in a separate container to make sure your salad doesn't wilt.

LUNCH

BLT SWEET POTATO TOAST
(Makes 1 serving)

◆ Meet your new favorite sandwich swap! Sweet potato subs in for the bread in this easy lunchtime classic.

TOTAL TIME: **15 MINUTES** / PREP TIME: **5 MINUTES** / COOKING TIME: **10 MINUTES**

---

2 ¼ inch thick slices sweet potato

2 slices turkey bacon

2 tsp. NSA mayonnaise

1 tomato, sliced

4 small pieces romaine lettuce

1. Coat sweet potato slices with cooking spray and place in toaster or on the rack in your toaster oven on highest setting.

2. Toast sweet potatoes 2–3 times, flipping each time for even browning, until cooked through.

3. While sweet potatoes toast, place bacon on a paper towel–lined microwave-safe plate and cover with paper towel.

4. Microwave on high for 3–4 minutes or until crispy.

5. Spread 1 tsp. mayonnaise on each slice of sweet potato toast.

6. Top with lettuce, tomato, and bacon.

TIPS

▶ Try to find mayonnaise made with avocado oil or olive oil. Bonus points if you make your own.

▶ Stir a little hot sauce into the mayonnaise for a delicious sweet-spicy riff on this dish.

DINNER

LEMON-THYME SHEET PAN ROAST CHICKEN
with Shallots & Carrots
(Makes 1 serving)

◆ This comfort-food supper cooks up to perfection in one sheet pan. Juicy chicken thighs are paired with a tangle of naturally sweet roasted carrots for a seriously delectable dinner.

TOTAL TIME: **25 MINUTES** / PREP TIME: **5 MINUTES** / COOKING TIME: **20 MINUTES**

6 oz. boneless skinless chicken thigh

2 cups carrots or rainbow carrots, peeled and cut into long, thin wedges

2 shallots or 1 small red onion, cut into wedges

1 Tbsp. fresh thyme (or 1 tsp. dried), additional for garnish

1 tsp. olive oil

1 tsp. lemon juice, additional lemon for serving

Fresh parsley for garnish (optional)

1. Preheat oven or toaster oven to 450 degrees and coat a small baking dish with cooking spray.

2. Place chicken on one side of pan and vegetables on the other side.

3. Sprinkle thyme, olive oil, lemon juice, and salt and pepper (as desired) on top. Toss to coat.

4. Roast for 20 minutes or until chicken is cooked through.

5. Serve garnished with additional fresh thyme, optional chopped parsley, and a lemon wedge.

TIP

▶ If you can't find fresh thyme in the supermarket, rosemary or sage would make worthy substitutions.

DINNER

CLASSIC BEEF BURGER
with Sweet Potato Fries & Special Sauce

(Makes 1 serving)

◆ Get your burger fix in a healthier way. You'll love the accompanying special sauce for dipping and also on top of burgers or sandwiches.

TOTAL TIME: **30 MINUTES** / PREP TIME: **5 MINUTES** / COOKING TIME: **25 MINUTES**

½ *large sweet potato, cut into ¼" wedges or French fry shapes*

1 tsp. olive oil

4 oz. 96% lean ground beef

Lettuce and tomato for serving (optional)

Special Sauce

1½ Tbsp. NSA mayonnaise

1 Tbsp. chopped dill pickle

1½ tsp. NSA ketchup

2 tsp. minced red onion

¼ tsp. Dijon mustard

Dash hot sauce

1. Preheat oven or toaster oven to 450 degrees.
2. Line a small baking pan with parchment.
3. Toss sweet potatoes in olive oil and season with salt and pepper (if desired).
4. Roast sweet potatoes for 20 minutes, stirring once, until well browned.
5. Mix together all Special Sauce ingredients in a small bowl and set aside.
6. Gently shape beef into a patty and season with salt and pepper (if desired).
7. Grill or pan fry burger on high heat until cooked to your liking (4–5 minutes per side for medium-rare).
8. Serve burger on lettuce and tomato with Special Sauce and sweet potato fries.

TIPS

▶ Parchment paper creates a nonstick surface and helps absorb moisture for a deliciously crispy, well-browned finish to your veggies.

▶ Be sure to checkout our **SF3** ketchup recipe, page 136.

DINNER

GRILLED CHICKEN PAILLARD
with Red Wine Vinaigrette over Arugula
(Makes 1 serving)

◆ This dish is perfect for busy weeknights! A juicy seasoned chicken cutlet tops a simple arugula and tomato salad. Try adding roasted or fresh sliced red peppers for even more color and crunch.

TOTAL TIME: **15 MINUTES** / PREP TIME: **5 MINUTES** / COOK TIME: **10 MINUTES**

5 oz. raw chicken breast cutlet (or raw boneless, skinless chicken breast)

1½ tsp. olive oil, divided

1½ tsp. Italian seasoning blend, divided

½ tsp. granulated garlic or garlic powder

3 cups baby arugula

1 cup grape or cherry tomatoes

1 tsp. red wine vinegar

1 tsp. Dijon mustard

1 small shallot, finely chopped

1 medium sweet potato

TIP

▶ Feel free to swap in other dark leafy greens such as baby spinach, baby kale, torn escarole, or romaine lettuce.

1. If chicken is not yet sliced into a cutlet, lay chicken breast on a cutting board, place one hand flat on top of the chicken and, holding a knife parallel to the cutting board, begin to slice it in half horizontally, but do not slice it completely in half. Open the sliced chicken like a book so that there is one large, flat, thin piece. If some parts are thicker than others, pound the thicker parts with a meat tenderizer or the back of a skillet.

2. Brush chicken with ½ tsp. olive oil and sprinkle with 1 tsp. Italian seasoning blend, garlic powder, salt, and pepper.

3. Heat grill or grill pan over high heat. Grill chicken for 3–4 minutes per side or until cooked through.

4. In a small bowl, whisk together remaining 1 tsp. olive oil, vinegar, mustard, shallot, and remaining ½ tsp. Italian seasoning blend.

5. Drizzle vinaigrette mixture over arugula, top with chicken and halved tomatoes. Season to taste with salt and pepper and serve immediately with a baked or mashed sweet potato.

DINNER

GRILLED FLANK STEAK
with Onions & Asparagus
(Makes 1 serving)

◆ Juicy, tender flank steak makes any weeknight feel more special! Here we serve it with tender asparagus and sweet grilled onions for a simple but satisfying meal.

TOTAL TIME: **20 MINUTES** / PREP TIME: **10 MINUTES** / COOKING TIME: **10 MINUTES**

---

4 oz. flank steak

¼ tsp. kosher salt

¼ tsp. granulated garlic

Pinch black pepper

½ red onion, thickly sliced

8 oz. asparagus spears, ends trimmed

½ tsp. olive oil

Cooking spray

TIP
▶ Double the steak in this recipe to use to top a salad for lunch the next day!

1. Season steak on both sides with salt, garlic, and pepper.

2. Place onion and asparagus in a large bowl and drizzle with olive oil.

3. Season vegetables with salt and pepper, to taste (as desired).

4. Coat a grill or large grill pan with cooking spray and heat over high heat.

5. Add steak and vegetables to heated grill.

6. Grill steak for 3–4 minutes per side for medium-rare or until cooked to your liking.

7. Grill vegetables for 5–7 minutes, turning occasionally, until lightly browned.

8. Let steak rest on a plate for 5 minutes before slicing crosswise against the grain.

9. Serve sliced steak and vegetables.

DINNER

SALMON WITH HERB PUREE
& Roasted Brussels Sprouts
(Makes 1 serving)

◆ A bright and flavorful mix of fresh herbs and tart lemon gives an amazing flavor boost to juicy roasted salmon.

TOTAL TIME: **25 MINUTES** / PREP TIME: **5 MINUTES** / COOKING TIME: **20 MINUTES**

---

2 cups brussels sprouts, halved if small, quartered if large

1 tsp. olive oil, divided

6 oz. salmon filet

⅛ tsp. garlic powder

Herb Puree

⅓ cup fresh chopped dill

⅓ cup fresh chopped parsley

1 scallion, chopped

1 tsp. dijon mustard

1 tsp. olive oil

1 Tbsp. warm water

2 tsp. lemon juice

1. Preheat your oven or toaster oven to 450 degrees and line a small baking dish with foil or parchment paper.

2. Toss brussels sprouts with ½ tsp. olive oil, season with salt and pepper (as desired), place on one side of prepared pan and roast for 10 minutes.

3. Brush salmon with remaining ½ tsp. olive oil and season with salt, pepper, and garlic powder. Place next to brussels sprouts and roast an additional 10 minutes for medium or to desired doneness.

4. Combine Herb Puree ingredients in a small food processor. Puree, scraping down the sides as needed, and season with salt and pepper to taste (as desired).

5. Serve salmon and roasted brussels sprouts drizzled with herb puree.

TIPS

▶ Roast two salmon filets at the same time to use the leftover for lunch!

▶ If you don't have a food processor to make the herb puree, you can finely chop all the ingredients and whisk together in a small bowl.

DINNER

EGG ROLL IN A BOWL
with Chicken or Shrimp
(Makes 1 serving)

◆ Enjoy all the flavors of your favorite egg roll in this lightened up one-pan dinner! Pre-made coleslaw mix slashes prep time, or use a mix of shredded cabbage and carrots.

TOTAL TIME: **15 MINUTES** / PREP TIME: **5 MINUTES** / COOKING TIME: **10 MINUTES**

2 tsp. sesame oil, divided

4 oz. thin sliced chicken breast or 4 oz. peeled deveined shrimp

3 scallions, sliced, green and white parts divided

2 cloves garlic, minced

1 tsp. fresh grated ginger

¼ cup sliced water chestnuts

4 cups coleslaw mix or mixed shredded cabbage and carrot

1½ tsp. soy sauce or tamari

1½ tsp. NSA rice wine vinegar

1 tsp. toasted sesame seeds

Chili-garlic sauce or cilantro for garnish (optional)

1. Heat 1 tsp. sesame oil in a large skillet over medium-high heat.

2. Add chicken or shrimp and stir fry for 3–4 minutes, stirring constantly, until cooked through.

3. Remove cooked chicken or shrimp to a plate. Set aside.

4. Add remaining 1 tsp. sesame oil to skillet and stir in white parts of scallion, garlic, and ginger. Cook for 1 minute.

5. Add water chestnuts, coleslaw mix, soy sauce, and rice wine vinegar. Cook, stirring frequently for 3–4 minutes or until vegetables are just wilted.

6. Add cooked chicken or shrimp back to pan, toss to combine, and season with salt and pepper.

7. Serve garnished with green parts of scallions and optional chili-garlic sauce, cilantro, and sesame seeds.

TIP

▶ This recipe is the perfect way to use up other bits of vegetables you may have on hand. Feel free to add mixed thin-sliced peppers, mushrooms, chopped broccoli, or baby spinach to the coleslaw mix.

DINNER

BROILED LEMON GARLIC SHRIMP
with Quinoa, Tomatoes & Spinach
(Makes 1 serving)

◆ Lightly seasoned shrimp top a filling, lemony quinoa pilaf in this easy weeknight supper.

TOTAL TIME: **25 MINUTES** / PREP TIME: **5 MINUTES** / COOKING TIME: **20 MINUTES**

---

6 oz. large shrimp, peeled and deveined

2 tsp. olive oil, divided

2 tsp. lemon juice, divided

¼ cup uncooked quinoa (or ½ cup pre-cooked quinoa)

½ tsp. lemon zest

2 minced garlic cloves

4 cups baby spinach

1 cup halved grape or cherry tomatoes

Torn fresh basil, hot pepper flakes, lemon wedge for garnish (optional)

1. Toss shrimp with 1 tsp. olive oil, 1 tsp. lemon juice, and a pinch of salt (if desired).

2. Place shrimp on a foil-lined baking pan and broil on high for 3–4 minutes or until pink and firm.

3. Cook quinoa according to package instructions and stir in remaining 1 tsp. olive oil, 1 tsp. lemon juice, minced clove garlic, ½ tsp. lemon zest, ¼ tsp. kosher salt, and baby spinach.

4. Stir to combine, cover, and cook 1 minute more to wilt spinach and so flavors combine.

5. Stir in tomatoes and serve quinoa topped with shrimp and garnished with optional basil, hot pepper flakes, and a squeeze of fresh lemon.

TIPS

▶ Seek out pre-cooked quinoa in the freezer or prepared food section to speed prep!

▶ Feel free to swap in other greens for the spinach such as baby kale, arugula, or Swiss chard.

BONUS DINNER

TURKEY ZUCCHINI PIZZA BOATS
(Makes 1 serving)

◆ Satisfy your pizza cravings with this unique dish! Tender broiled zucchini is stuffed with a savory garlicky turkey marinara filling and topped with melty cheese for a filling and fun dinner.

TOTAL TIME: **24 MINUTES** / PREP TIME: **5 MINUTES** / COOKING TIME: **19 MINUTES**

Olive oil cooking spray

4 oz. lean ground turkey

⅓ cup minced onion

2 tsp. minced garlic

¾ cup NSA marinara, divided

1 medium zucchini, halved lengthwise and seeds scooped out

½ tsp. garlic salt

3 Tbsp. part-skim shredded mozzarella cheese

2 tsp. grated parmesan cheese

2 Tbsp. chopped basil

1. Coat a medium non-stick sauté pan with cooking spray and heat over medium-high heat.

2. Add turkey and onion and cook, stirring frequently and breaking up turkey with a wooden spoon for 5 minutes or until turkey is no longer pink.

3. Stir in garlic and cook for 1 minute.

4. Stir in ½ cup of marinara, turn off the heat, and set aside.

5. Preheat oven or toaster oven to 450 degrees and line a small baking pan with foil.

6. Place zucchini boats cut side up on pan, spray with cooking spray, and sprinkle with garlic salt.

7. Roast zucchini for 10 minutes or until fork tender.

8. Fill zucchini with turkey mixture, sprinkle with mozzarella and parmesan cheeses, and return to oven to melt cheese and heat through for 3 minutes.

9. Serve garnished with basil and with remaining ¼ cup marinara for dipping.

TIP

▶ You can make the turkey mixture up to 3 days ahead to speed dinner prep.

CONDIMENTS, SAUCES & DRESSINGS

SF3 KETCHUP
(Makes 1¾ cups ketchup)

 Vegan

◆ Skip the sugary ketchup and whip up a batch of our super flavorful **SF3** version instead!

TOTAL TIME: **25 MINUTES** / PREP TIME: **5 MINUTES** / COOKING TIME: **20 MINUTES**

---

8 oz. can tomato sauce

6 oz. can tomato paste

¾ cup water

1½ Tbsp. apple cider vinegar

1 Tbsp soy sauce

½ tsp. onion powder

¼ tsp. garlic powder

Pinch allspice

Salt to taste

Stevia or monk fruit to taste (optional, as desired)

1. Combine all ingredients in a small saucepan and simmer over medium-low heat for 20 minutes to slightly reduce.

2. Season to taste with salt, pepper, and optional stevia or monk fruit.

TIP
▶ **SF3** Ketchup will keep in the refrigerator for up to a week in an air-tight container to enjoy with eggs, roasted veggies, or on burgers.

CONDIMENTS, SAUCES & DRESSINGS

SF3 BBQ SAUCE
(Makes 1 cup)

 Vegan

◆ Most barbecue sauces are sugar bombs but not our **SF3** version! Brush this thick, smoky sauce on grilled chicken or enjoy it to top burgers too!

TOTAL TIME: **25 MINUTES** / PREP TIME: **5 MINUTES** / COOKING TIME: **20 MINUTES**

6 oz. can tomato paste
2 Tbsp. apple cider vinegar
1 Tbsp. soy sauce
1 tsp. smoked paprika
1 tsp. onion powder
½ tsp. garlic powder
½ tsp. kosher salt
¼ tsp. chili powder
Stevia or monk fruit, optional as desired

1. Combine all ingredients in a small saucepan.
2. Add ½ cup water and simmer over low heat for 20 minutes for flavors to combine.
3. Season with optional stevia or monk fruit for sweetness.

TIP
▶ Give your **SF3** Barbecue sauce a kick by adding a bit of cayenne pepper or hot sauce.

CONDIMENTS, SAUCES & DRESSINGS

SF3 MARINARA SAUCE
(Makes 2½ cups or 4 servings)

 Vegan

◆ Get your Italian food fix with our flavor-packed tomato sauce! It will be your go-to to top zucchini noodles, grilled veggies, or even Italian omelettes for breakfast.

TOTAL TIME: **30 MINUTES** / PREP TIME: **5 MINUTES** / COOKING TIME: **25 MINUTES**

---

1 Tbsp. olive oil

½ cup chopped onion

1 Tbsp. kosher salt, divided

¼ tsp. red chili flakes

2 tsp. minced garlic

1 35 oz. can crushed San Marzano tomatoes in juice

¼ cup minced fresh basil

1 tsp. no-salt Italian seasoning

1. Heat olive oil in a large soup pot or dutch oven over medium-low heat.

2. Add onions and sprinkle with 1 tsp. salt.

3. Cook, stirring often, until golden and softened, about 10–15 minutes.

4. Add chili flakes and garlic and cook for 1 minute.

5. Add tomatoes, basil, Italian seasoning, remaining 2 tsp. salt to pot. Bring to a simmer, stirring often, and cook for an additional 10 minutes for flavors to meld.

TIP

▶ This SF3 marinara sauce freezes really well, so make a double batch to keep on hand in the freezer for busy weeknights!

CONDIMENTS, SAUCES & DRESSINGS

CREAMY RANCH DRESSING
(Makes 6 servings)

◆ This **SF3** ranch has amazing flavor thanks to a mix of fresh herbs, while the Greek yogurt gives it a boost of protein . Enjoy it to top salads or as an easy dip with crudités.

TOTAL TIME: **5 MINUTES** / PREP TIME: **5 MINUTES** / COOKING TIME: **0 MINUTES**

---

1 cup Greek yogurt (2%)

2 Tbsp. water

1 tsp. minced garlic

1 Tbsp. minced fresh dill

1 Tbsp. minced fresh parsley

1 Tbsp. chopped scallion

¼ tsp. cider vinegar

1. Whisk together all ingredients and keep chilled in an air-tight container in the refrigerator for up to 1 week.

TIPS

▶ Swap in other soft herbs you have on hand such as cilantro, tarragon, or mint to give your ranch a different twist.

▶ You can also use slightly less water if you want a thicker ranch dip for veggies.

CONDIMENTS, SAUCES & DRESSINGS

CREAMY TAHINI DRIZZLE
(Yields 1 cup to serve 8)

◆ This super flavorful, highly addictive tahini dressing will become your favorite salad drizzle, dip for crudités, or topping for grilled or roasted veggies.

TOTAL TIME: **5 MINUTES** / PREP TIME: **5 MINUTES** / COOKING TIME: **0 MINUTES**

⅓ cup tahini

⅓ cup Greek yogurt (2%)

¼ cup warm water, additional as needed

2 tsp. lemon juice

1 tsp. minced garlic

½ tsp. cumin

½ tsp. kosher salt

¼ tsp. smoked paprika

1. Whisk all ingredients together in a small bowl (adding more water if needed to thin).

TIP

▶ Tahini is made from pureed sesame seeds and is a great peanut butter swap for those with nut allergies. You can find it by the peanut butter or in the international section of most major supermarkets.

DESSERTS

EASY CINNAMON "BAKED" APPLES
(Makes 1 serving)

 Vegan

◆ Enjoy all the flavor of apple pie in this so-simple microwave dessert!

TOTAL TIME: **7 MINUTES** / PREP TIME: **5 MINUTES** / COOKING TIME: **2 MINUTES**

*1 Honeycrisp or
Macoun Apple,
cut into 12 wedges*

¼ tsp. water

¼ tsp. cinnamon

*1 Tbsp. toasted
chopped pecans*

1. Combine apple wedges, water, and cinnamon in a small microwaveable bowl.

2. Cover bowl with a wet paper towel or wax paper and vent to let steam escape

3. Microwave on high for 2 minutes. Let cool for 1 minute.

4. Top with pecans.

TIPS

▶ Feel free to sprinkle a little nutmeg or cardamon!

▶ Make 2–3 at a time.

▶ Puree for apple sauce.

▶ Top a pancake.

DESERTS

ROASTED CHERRIES
with Whipped Ricotta and Walnuts
(Makes 2 servings)

◆ You won't believe how easy it is to make this decadent-seeming dessert! Frozen cherries are transformed into a thick, rich topping for fluffy ricotta.

TOTAL TIME: **25 MINUTES** / PREP TIME: **5 MINUTES** / COOKING TIME: **20 MINUTES**

10 oz. bag defrosted frozen cherries (2 cups)

½ tsp. cornstarch

¼ tsp. vanilla extract

½ cup part-skim ricotta cheese

2 Tbsp. toasted chopped walnuts

1. Preheat oven or toaster oven to 450°F.

2. Line an 8x8 baking pan with aluminum foil; lightly coat with cooking spray.

3. Spread cherries on prepared pan and stir in cornstarch.

4. Roast, stirring once, until wilted and juices are starting to brown or about 20 minutes.

5. Spoon roasted cherries and juices into a bowl; stir in vanilla.

6. Beat ricotta with an electric beater in a small bowl until fluffy.

7. Serve ricotta topped with cherries and garnished with walnuts.

TIPS

▶ Add a pinch of nutmeg or cardamom to the cherries for a fun flavor twist.

▶ Cherries can be served with NSA yogurt or over our pancakes.

DESSERTS

WATERMELON MINT GRANITA

(Makes 2 servings)

 Vegan

◆ Our easy frozen treat is inspired by tropical mojitos! Naturally sweet and juicy watermelon makes the perfect **SF3** dessert.

TOTAL TIME: **1½ HOURS**, LARGELY UNATTENDED
PREP TIME: **5 MINUTES** / COOKING TIME: **0 MINUTES**

---

3 cups cubed watermelon

2 tsp. lime juice

1 Tbsp. chopped fresh mint

1. Place watermelon and lime juice in a blender or food processor and blend to a puree.

2. Stir in fresh mint.

3. Pour watermelon mixture into a loaf pan and place in the freezer.

4. Scrape the frozen corners of the pan to the center every 30–40 minutes or until mixture is fully frozen and fluffy.

5. Serve in a small bowl or a cup.

TIPS

▶ If your granita freezes all the way through, just pulse in a blender or mini chop to a snow-cone texture.

▶ Feel free to swap in ripe, juicy cantaloupe or honeydew melon, if you prefer.

WILLING TO COOK

This 7-day plan requires less meal prep and uses pre-washed and pre-cooked foods for a fast and easy approach.

Even though the recipes are delicious and some people love to cook, not everyone has time to make recipes from scratch. That's why I love this approach because I still have complete control of what I'm eating without all the legwork. And with the label-reading knowledge in Chapter 3, it's never been easier.

	BREAKFAST	LUNCH	DINNER
Monday	Protein shake	Build a bowl	Simply grilled
Tuesday	Protein shake	Build a bowl +	1 Pan roast
Wednesday	Egg sandwich	Quick salad	Simple foil bake
Thursday	Yogurt parfait	Quick salad +	Burger night
Friday	Yogurt parfait +	Sandwich	Pasta night
Saturday	Easy oatmeal	Soup	Kebobs
Sunday	Easy oatmeal +	Wrap	Stirfry

BREAKFAST

PROTEIN SHAKE: 1 serving of fruit, 1 cup unsweetened almond milk, 1 scoop NSA protein powder, 1 tbsp. nut butter, ice, and blend in blender.

EGG SANDWICH: 2 eggs any style (+ opt. veggies, cheese, or avocado) on NSA **SF3**-approved toast.

YOGURT PARFAIT: 2% plain or NSA Greek yogurt + nuts or nut butter (opt. fruit).

YOGURT PARFAIT+: 2% plain or NSA Greek yogurt + nuts or nut butter + fruit of choice (cinammon, extracts optional).

EASY OATMEAL: Oatmeal + toasted nuts or nut butter + berries.

EASY OATMEAL+: Oatmeal + nuts or nut butter + berries (opt. milk or plant-based milk, opt. cinnamon).

LUNCH

BUILD A BOWL: Pick at least 2 veggies (prewashed and chopped or frozen), pick your pre-cooked protein (chicken, shrimp or egg), pick the grain or bean and marinade or sauce of your choice.

BUILD A BOWL+: Pick at least 2 veggies (prewashed and chopped), pre-cooked protein, pick your grain, + cheese or avocado, fresh salsa, marinade or sauce of your choice.

QUICK SALAD: Prewashed lettuce (arugula, spinach, or mix) + pre-cooked protein + NSA dressing + avocado.

QUICK SALAD+: Prewashed lettuce (arugula, spinach, or mix) + veggies + pre-cooked protein + NSA dressing (+beans, nuts, avocado and/or cheese).

SANDWICH: Pick an NSA approved bread or go bunless, add cooked protein like turkey breast, chicken, or turkey burger, tomato, lettuce, avocado, and dressing of your choice.

SOUP: Chicken, veggie, or beef based broth with veggies, beans, or approved noodles + a fruit.

WRAP: Pick an NSA **SF3**-approved wrap. Pick at least 2 veggies, pick your protein, + cheese or avocado, salsa, mustard + sauce of your choice.

DINNER

SIMPLY GRILLED: Select lean steak, turkey, or chicken burger, chicken cutlet, fish, or seafood and lightly coat with a little olive oil, salt, pepper, or favorite seasoning or marinade and grill up! + Pair with grilled veggies or salad+ opt. baked or roast potato.

1 PAN ROAST: Brush piece of chicken, steak, or fish with olive oil, salt, and pepper or favorite marinade . Toss veggies of your choice with a little olive oil, salt, and pepper. Roast in oven at 325–350 degrees for chicken, 400–450 degrees for fish, 375 degrees for meat.

SIMPLE FOIL BAKE: Great for "steam-like" plain fish or seafood (or any protein): brush protein with olive oil, lemon, salt and pepper or favorite rub or marinade and wrap in foil and bake for 30 minutes at 350–375 degrees. Serve with salad or 2 veggie + opt. grain or potato.

BURGER NIGHT: 1–2 Trader Joe's or other premade chicken, turkey, or beef burger patty. Bake, grill or broil as per package. Enjoy with salad, tomato, onion, pickle, avocado and/or favorite veggie and baked potato or baked potato fries or **SF3**-approved rub.

PASTA NIGHT: Select whole wheat pasta, bean pasta, or favorite **SF3**-approved pasta. Add pre-cooked protein, add 1–2 fresh or frozen veggies and NSA sauce of your choice (marinara, garlic and olive oil, pesto).

KEBOBS: Select steak, chicken, fish + skewer with veggies like mushroom, peppers, and onion (season as needed with olive oil, salt, and pepper). Grill and serve over rice and sauce of your choice (hummus, tahini, Asian or Italian).

STIRFRY: Select steak, chicken, or shrimp. Sauté your favorite frozen veggies in pan with a little oil (garlic or onion if desired). Add in pre-cooked protein, toss with salt, pepper. Season with soy sauce, broth if needed. Serve over brown or cauliflower rice.

Fast & Easy 12-Minute Recipes.
If you're busy like me, you'll probably love these 12 recipes on the following pages— all 12 minutes or less.

BREAKFAST

AVOCADO TOAST WITH EGG
(Makes 1 serving)

◆ This speedy and satisfying toast gets a great protein boost from a luscious egg topper!

TOTAL TIME: **10 MINUTES** / PREP TIME: **5 MINUTES** / COOKING TIME: **5 MINUTES**

⅓ ripe avocado, mashed

½ tsp. lemon juice

1 slice NSA whole grain bread, toasted

1 large egg

1 tsp. chopped chives

Olive oil cooking spray

1. Combine avocado, lemon juice, and a pinch of salt in a small bowl.

2. Spread avocado mixture on top of toast.

3. Coat a small nonstick sauté pan with cooking spray and heat over medium-high heat.

4. Fry egg until done to your liking, 3–4 minutes for sunny side up or flip halfway through cooking and cook for an additional 1–2 minutes for over easy or over hard.

5. Serve avocado toast topped with egg, seasoned with optional salt and pepper, and garnished with chives.

TIP

▶ Try garnishing your toast with minced onion, hot sauce, or other chopped fresh herbs such as parsley, basil, or dill.

BREAKFAST

SMOKED SALMON TOAST
(Makes 1 serving)

◆ This brunch bistro classic is easy to make at home! Smoked salmon is a great source of protein and healthy omega-3s and a delicious topper for your favorite avo toast.

TOTAL TIME: **5 MINUTES** / PREP TIME: **5 MINUTES** / COOKING TIME: **0 MINUTES**

⅓ ripe avocado, mashed

½ tsp. lemon juice

1 slice NSA whole grain bread, toasted

2 oz. sliced smoked salmon

1 tsp. minced red onion or shallot

1 tsp. chopped fresh dill

1. Combine avocado, lemon juice, and a pinch of salt in a small bowl.

2. Spread avocado mixture on top of toast and top with smoked salmon, onion, and dill.

TIP
▶ For a flavor boost try adding capers and tomato.

BREAKFAST

RICOTTA & PEACH BREAKFAST TOAST
(Makes 1 serving)

◆ Satisfy your sweet tooth with this fun and healthy take on a fruit and cheese danish! Creamy ricotta cheese is delicious topped with juicy peaches or other fresh fruit.

TOTAL TIME: **5 MINUTES** / PREP TIME: **5 MINUTES** / COOKING TIME: **0 MINUTES**

---

1 slice NSA whole grain bread, toasted

¼ cup part-skim ricotta cheese

⅓ cup frozen peach slices, defrosted and halved

1 tsp. chopped fresh mint

1. Spread ricotta cheese on toast and top with peach slices and mint.

TIP

▶ I love using frozen peaches for this recipe because they're available year round and always juicy and sweet. Feel free to swap in fresh peaches or nectarines in season.

BREAKFAST

CINNAMON SPICE OATMEAL
with Toasted Pecans
(Makes 1 serving)

 Vegan

◆ This lightly spiced, creamy, satisfying oatmeal will be your go-to on busy mornings! Add toasted pecans for delicious crunch.

TOTAL TIME: **11 MINUTES** / PREP TIME: **5 MINUTES** / COOKING TIME: **6 MINUTES**

½ cup old-fashioned oats

1 cup vanilla unsweetened almond milk

½ tsp. cinnamon

1 Tbsp. chopped toasted pecans

1. Combine oats, almond milk, and cinnamon in a small microwaveable bowl.

2. Cover bowl with plastic wrap or wax paper and microwave on medium power for 5 minutes.

3. Uncover, stir, and let cool for 1 minute before eating.

4. Garnish with pecans and enjoy.

TIP

▶ Add bananas or berries for natural sweetness.

LUNCH OR DINNER

VEGAN MISO SOUP
with Tofu & Veggies
(Makes 1 serving)

 Vegan

◆ You won't believe how easy it is to make your own miso soup at home! This version features a hearty mix of tofu, Swiss chard, shiitakes, and bean sprouts for a filling and flavorful bowl.

TOTAL TIME: **10 MINUTES** / PREP TIME: **5 MINUTES** / COOKING TIME: **5 MINUTES**

2 cups vegetable broth

1 sheet nori (dried seaweed) cut into small squares

2 Tbsp. white miso paste

½ cup chopped Swiss chard or other dark leafy green

¼ cup sliced shiitake mushrooms

¼ cup chopped scallions

⅓ cup extra firm tofu, cubed

¼ cup bean sprouts

½ tsp. NSA rice vinegar

1. Place vegetable broth in a medium sauce pan and bring to a low simmer.

2. Add nori and simmer, uncovered, for 5–7 minutes.

3. While broth simmers, place miso into a small bowl and whisk in a little hot water until smooth.

4. Add Swiss chard, shiitakes, green onion, tofu, and sprouts to the simmering broth and cook for 5 minutes.

5. Remove pot from the heat, stir in miso mixture and rice vinegar, and enjoy.

TIP

▶ Give this soup a spicy kick by stirring in some chili-garlic sauce at the end.

LUNCH OR DINNER

VIETNAMESE TURKEY LETTUCE WRAPS
with Cucumber-Peanut Relish
(Makes 1 serving)

◆ Lightly spiced sautéed ground turkey is tucked into wraps and topped with a crunchy topping for a fun and delicious lunch.

TOTAL TIME: **12 MINUTES** / PREP TIME: **5 MINUTES** / COOKING TIME: **7 MINUTES**

Filling

- ¼ lb. lean ground turkey
- 2 large scallions, chopped
- 1 tsp. ginger
- 1 tsp. soy sauce
- 1 tsp. NSA rice vinegar
- 1 tsp. sesame oil
- 3 large Boston lettuce leaves

Olive oil cooking spray

Relish

- ¼ cup diced cucumber
- ¼ cup diced red pepper
- 1 scallion, chopped
- 2 Tbsp. combined chopped cilantro and mint
- 1 Tbsp. chopped toasted peanuts

1. Coat a medium nonstick sauté pan with cooking spray and heat over medium-high heat.

2. Add turkey, scallion, and ginger and cook for 5–7 minutes, stirring frequently and breaking the turkey up with a wooden spoon, until no longer pink.

3. Stir soy sauce and rice vinegar into turkey mixture and keep warm,

4. Toss together all relish ingredients in a small bowl.

5. Serve turkey mixture tucked into lettuce leaves, topped with relish, and drizzled with sesame oil.

TIP

▶ This dish can be made ahead! Just rewarm the turkey mixture and assemble your wraps right before eating.

LUNCH OR DINNER

STEAK TACO GRAIN BOWL
with Avocado
(Makes 1 serving)

◆ This hearty and substantial recipe makes a fantastic weekday lunch. Enjoy all the flavors of your favorite burrito in a lightened up, easy-to-eat bowl!

TOTAL TIME: **5 MINUTES** / PREP TIME: **5 MINUTES** / COOKING TIME: **0 MINUTES**

2 Tbsp. Greek yogurt (2% fat)

¼ tsp. lime zest

4 oz. sliced grilled flank steak

½ cup chopped baby spinach

¼ cup cooked brown rice

¼ cup canned black beans, rinsed and drained

½ cup diced yellow pepper

¼ sliced avocado

2 Tbsp. salsa

2 Tbsp. light shredded cheddar cheese

1. Whisk together yogurt and lime zest.
2. Add steak, spinach, rice, and beans to the bottom of another bowl.
3. Top with pepper, avocado, salsa, and cheese.
4. Dollop with yogurt and enjoy.

TIP

▶ This recipe is the perfect way to use up leftover steak from dinner the night before. You can also swap in leftover grilled chicken, pork, or shrimp, if you like.

LUNCH OR DINNER

SHREDDED CHICKEN GYRO BOWL
with Creamy Tahini Drizzle
(Makes 1 serving)

◆ Give your basic chicken-topped salad a fun new twist in this Mediterranean inspired bowl! A mix of veggies, chickpeas, and a luscious sesame-flavored tahini sauce make this salad special.

TOTAL TIME: **5 MINUTES** / PREP TIME: **5 MINUTES** / COOKING TIME: **0 MINUTES**

1½ cups baby spinach or baby kale

4 oz. shredded cooked chicken

½ cup canned chickpeas, rinsed and drained

¼ cup diced cucumber

¼ cup halved cherry or grape tomatoes

2 Tbsp. minced red onion

2 Tbsp. Creamy Tahini Drizzle (see page 140)

1 Tbsp. chopped fresh mint (optional, as desired)

1. Place spinach, chicken, and chickpeas in a large serving bowl.

2. Top with cucumber, tomato, and red onion.

3. Drizzle with tahini sauce and garnish with optional torn mint.

TIP

▶ Make a batch of Creamy Tahini Drizzle to use for this recipe, enjoy as a veggie dip, or to top grilled or roasted vegetables.

LUNCH OR DINNER

MEDITERRANEAN PLATTER
with Pickled Veggies & Tahini Drizzle
(Makes 1 serving)

◆ The fun mix of flavors, colors, and textures in this platter is sure to make your tastebuds happy! Keep a variety of NSA pickled veggies on hand to add tang and crunch to all your salads and bowl recipes.

TOTAL TIME: **5 MINUTES** / PREP TIME: **5 MINUTES** / COOKING TIME: **0 MINUTES**

⅔ cup canned chickpeas, rinsed and drained

1 cup baby spinach, baby kale, or arugula

½ cup jarred, NSA pickled vegetables, drained

⅓ cup diced bell pepper

⅓ cup diced tomato or halved grape tomatoes

⅓ cup diced cucumber

3 Tbsp. prepared hummus

2 Tbsp. Creamy Tahini Drizzle (see page 140)

2 Tbsp. chopped fresh mint

1. Arrange chickpeas, greens, pickled vegetables, mixed diced vegetables, and hummus on a large plate.

2. Drizzle chickpeas and vegetables with tahini sauce and garnish with fresh mint.

TIP
▶ This platter is a fantastic way to use up any leftover raw or cooked veggies you have on hand.

LUNCH OR DINNER

EASY CHICKEN CLUB LETTUCE WRAPS
(Makes 1 serving)

◆ Enjoy all the flavors of your favorite club sandwich in these easy lettuce wraps! Perfect for a speedy weekday lunch or light dinner.

TOTAL TIME: **8 MINUTES** / PREP TIME: **5 MINUTES** / COOKING TIME: **3 MINUTES**

1 slice turkey bacon

3 large Boston lettuce leaves

1 tsp. NSA mayonnaise

1 medium tomato, cut into 6 slices

4 oz. grilled chicken, sliced

¼ avocado, sliced

1. Place bacon on a paper towel–lined plate.
2. Cover with a paper towel and microwave for 2 minutes or until crisp. Crumble when cool.
3. Arrange lettuce leaves on a plate and top each with a dap of mayonnaise.
4. Top lettuce leaves evenly with tomato slices, chicken slices, avocado slices, and crumbled bacon. Enjoy!

TIPS

▶ Swap in any sturdy greens you have on hand such as romaine lettuce, Napa cabbage, or collard greens.

▶ Stir some hot sauce into your mayonnaise to give these wraps a little kick.

SIDES AND SNACKS

FRIED CAULI RICE
(Makes 1 serving)

 Vegan

◆ You won't miss the heavier takeout version when you try this lighter rendition of your favorite fried rice!

TOTAL TIME: **10 MINUTES** / PREP TIME: **5 MINUTES** / COOKING TIME: **5 MINUTES**

1 tsp. minced garlic
1 tsp. minced ginger
1¼ cups cauliflower rice
½ cup defrosted frozen peas and carrots
2 tsp. soy sauce
1 tsp. no-sugar rice vinegar
1 tsp. sesame oil
1 Tbsp. chopped scallion
Cooking spray

1. Coat a medium nonstick sauté pan with cooking spray and heat over medium heat.

2. Add garlic, ginger, cauliflower rice, peas and carrots to pan and cook for 3–4 minutes or until vegetables are tender but not soft.

3. Stir in soy sauce, rice vinegar, and sesame oil and serve garnished with chopped scallion.

TIPS

▶ Keep frozen cauliflower rice in the freezer to make this flavorful side dish anytime.

▶ Add chopped cooked egg, chicken, or shrimp for a complete meal.

SIDES AND SNACKS

CAPRESE STACKS
(Makes 1 serving)

◆ These adorable fresh mozzarella and tomato bites make the perfect anytime snack!

TOTAL TIME: **5 MINUTES** / PREP TIME: **5 MINUTES** / COOKING TIME: **0 MINUTES**

---

1 large plum tomato, sliced into 5 rounds

1½ oz. small fresh mozzarella balls (or bocconcini), cut into 5 pieces

½ tsp. olive oil

1 Tbsp. chopped fresh basil

Coarse ground pepper and sea salt, optional, as desired

1. Arrange tomato slices on a plate.
2. Top evenly with mozzarella.
3. Drizzle with olive oil, top with basil, and season as desired with salt and pepper.

TIP

▶ Try garnishing these stacks with minced scallion, chopped fresh mint, or chopped chives for a fun flavor twist.

DON'T COOK

Use this 7-day sample plan as a guide if you don't cook and will either order in, take out, or dine out.

Let's be honest, some of us are just too busy to grocery shop and prep meals, or our jobs require travel and we just have eat out. Here are some ideas to help keep you on track. These foods require minimal preparation or can easily be found in restaurants. Reference the dining out guide for more ideas.

	BREAKFAST	LUNCH	DINNER
Monday	Oatmeal and 2 hard-boiled eggs or eggs any way	Salad: Greek salad with choice of protein	Grilled or roast chicken with roast brussels sprouts and brown rice
Tuesday	Oatmeal and 2 hard-boiled eggs or eggs any way	Salad: chicken caesar salad	Beef burger with baked or sweet potato
Wednesday	Poached or scrambled eggs with avocado + fruit salad	Sandwich: Openface turkey sandwich, lettuce, tomato, avocado, mustard	Italian: Grilled fish with sautéed spinach, zoodles, garlic and olive oil
Thursday	Poached or scrambled eggs with avocado + fruit salad	Japanese: Sashimi, edamame, miso soup, and brown rice	Grilled steak with asparagus and baked potato
Friday	Fruit + plain Greek yogurt	American: Bunless burger with baked sweet potato with avocado + turkey bacon	Seafood: Grilled fish or shrimp with grilled veggies like asparagus
Saturday	Fruit + plain Greek yogurt	Grain bowl: Grain bowl with shrimp, veggies, black beans, avocado, salsa	Chinese: Steamed Chinese veggies, chicken or shrimp, and brown rice
Sunday	Egg and cheese with fruit or potato	Grain bowl: Quinoa with veggies and choice of protein	Asian: Poké bowl, brown rice, and green salad

CHAPTER

6

HOW TO MAXIMIZE WEIGHT LOSS

Nine Ways to Shed Extra Pounds
in the Healthiest Possible Way

I F LOSING WEIGHT is your top goal, you'll want to pay close attention to this chapter. For those of you who have had less than nutritious eating habits before starting the program— we're talking a diet that consisted of a lot of packaged, processed foods that are laden with added sugar—it's very possible that just following the basic principles will be enough of a shift to help you lose the unhealthy excess weight you've been carrying around.

But for those of you who, like me, eat pretty healthily and just want to reboot your system and ditch the junk in order to feel better, you may need to take some extra measures to lose a targeted amount of weight. What follows is advice on how to do that in a healthy and sustainable way.

I asked my friend Max Lugavere, author of *Genius Foods*, if there's a direct link between giving up added sugars and this kind of weight loss and gaining a feeling of control. He wrote me back with a resounding yes! "Giving up sugar can lead to weight loss because you're limiting the consumption of calorie-dense, nutrient-poor packaged, processed foods, which are usually the foods in the supermarket with added sugars," he told me. "Once you eliminate foods with added sugars—including commercial breads, sauces, fruit juices, yogurts, and even salad dressings—your hunger will much more naturally regulate itself so that you needn't rely on willpower, which is a finite and fragile resource! You'll end up eating less, naturally, which will lead to"—you guessed it—"weight loss."

Weight Loss Winners

Check out some of **Sugar Free 3**'s biggest losers from among those who tried it first!

JUDY G.	JUAN M.	BRUCE K.
Stay-at-Home Mom	Project Manager	Consultant
16 pounds	**13 pounds**	**13 pounds**

COURTNEE S.	JOSLYN B.	MICHAEL K.
Head Start Teacher	Marketing Manager	Self-Employed
11 pounds	**8.5 pounds**	**7.5 pounds**

By eliminating added sugars, you aren't losing anything you need to function optimally; you're just replacing empty calories with nutritious ones and that alone is helpful. "Giving up sugar helps with weight loss in many ways," says Keri Glassman, MS, RDN, CDN, and founder and CEO of the Nutritious Life Studio. "First of all, sugar equals extra calories, and extra calories eventually turn to fat to be stored if they aren't needed for fuel by the body. Secondly, sugar is easy to overconsume because, well, it tastes good!"

Even as a nutritionist, Keri is not immune to sugar's call. Her thing is chocolate—ideally, very dark chocolate, which does have some redeeming health properties. "We all have natural taste for sweet foods," Keri explains, "but because sugary foods lack fiber and protein most of the time, they don't keep you full or satisfied."

But just because there's no calorie or macro counting or portioning of food on **Sugar Free 3**, that doesn't mean you can graze all day. And if you really desire to slim down, you might even need to cut back on some of the allowable foods. Some tips:

Moderate Your Fruit

Fruit is good for you—"better than any refined sugar, because it's a whole food that comes with antioxidants and fiber, which helps regulate blood sugar," says Keri. But if weight loss is your goal, you should limit your servings to one to two servings a day, like a cup of berries or a small-to-medium-size apple. While the sugar is naturally occurring, some fruit contains 15–30 grams per serving depending on which you choose. So you definitely do not want to be drinking a smoothie loaded with four different fruits for breakfast. Because of its sweetness, fruit is great for fighting sugar cravings, but, cautions Keri, "for people who have a strong sugar addiction, or who want to lose weight, you can actually overindulge in grapes if you're eating them all day long."

Limit Grains and Starchy Veggies

Starches tend to be more caloric than many foods, and are sometimes easy to overeat. Limit even the **SF3**-approved brown rice, whole- and sprouted-grain breads, potatoes, and sweet potatoes to one to two servings a day.

Don't Go Nuts on Nuts

Personally, I found that when I cut sugar, I was tempted to eat more fats—and healthy fats are allowed on **Sugar Free 3**. Even so, you need to be mindful of how much you're consuming. Nuts are a great way to feel satisfied, but they are high in fat—and therefore calories—and people have a tendency to eat too much of them. I'm one of those people. Keep in mind that a tablespoon of nut butter is around 100 calories—and a lot more if it's a heaping scoop. A small handful of nuts is about 150 calories—and it's almost impossible not to grab them by the handful (that's not just me, right?). So even though portion control is not a foundational requirement of **SF3**, if you want to trim weight, you need to pay closer attention and not fall prey to mindless munching. I recommend that you portion out foods that you find harder to control your consumption of, and put the bag or jar back in the pantry before eating.

Stop Eating after Dinner

Hopefully, you're following the guidelines I've recommended in this book, including a balanced, healthy breakfast, lunch, and dinner and

INSIDER SECRET

▶ Brush your teeth after every meal. You'll be less likely to pop something into a fresh, minty mouth.

maybe a snack or two. If you're eating like this, you should have all the food you need for the day, so continued snacking will only mean unneeded calories.

That said, nightly snacking habits are tough to beat—especially sugary ones. If it's late and you're really craving something sweet—and none of the tips I share in Chapter 8 are quelling the urge—don't cave in! Sometimes a simple piece of fruit will suffice. "If it's between a candy bar and a piece of fruit, obviously go for the piece of fruit," says Keri.

Track Your Intake

There is research to suggest that tracking what you consume helps you eat less. Use a food journal (there's a sample in the Appendix), the Openfit app, or even the notes section on your phone. Things to track to reach your weight-loss goal include:

- *What you eat for each meal*
- *Your fruit, grains, and starchy veggies (note them separately)*
- *How much water you drink*
- *Cravings*
- *Sleep quality and hours*
- *How you feel*
- *Your weight*

Drink More Water

Aim for your weight divided by two in ounces. So if you weigh 200 pounds, that's 100 ounces of water, or 12½ 8-ounce glasses. Drink more if you're working out or have headaches or cravings. You'll feel fuller faster.

Get Moving

Exercise has so many benefits—you'll be in a better mood, have bonus energy, and of course, kicking up a sweat helps with weight loss. So grab your sneaks and get after it! Try a walk, a jog, a hike, an indoor cycling class, or an online workout like those on Openfit.

Measure Pounds and Inches

If you want to monitor your progress on the scale, that's fine. A weekly check-in is a good way to gauge progress. But you might also want to measure the inches around your waist, thighs, chest, and upper arms. (Make sure to measure the exact same spot every time!) This will give you some perspective, especially if you exercise, because your body can transform in a positive way even if the scale doesn't budge. Remember, muscle weighs more than fat, by volume; its density can make the circumference smaller. Besides, lean tissue burns more calories, even at rest. "I have done **Sugar Free 3** twice—and I've lost almost 25 pounds after the two rounds," said Juan M., an Openfit project manager, who was motivated by measuring. "I have not been this weight in over 4 years! I have gone down at least one notch on my belt and my clothes are feeling much looser."

Avoid the "Barely Allowed" Section

The foods on the "Barely Allowed" list are high in fat and calories, so sidestep them to achieve your weight loss goals.

Ditch the Mindful Indulgence

You won't be counting calories on **Sugar Free 3**. But the more calories you eat, the harder it is to lose weight. To maximize the plan for weight loss, just say no to your Mindful Indulgence.

Controversial Topic: How Often Should You Weigh Yourself? Understandably, some people fear the scale or avoid it because they find it leads to obsessive thinking or unhealthy behavior. If that's you, then stay away! But if more frequent weigh-ins help you focus on your goals and behavior, then it's fine to do, according to registered dietitian Keri Glassman.

CHAPTER

7

DINING OUT AND OTHER SOCIAL SITUATIONS

Coping Advice for the Times
You're Not in Total Control of Your Food

PERSONALLY, I'VE NEVER had a three-week period where I could lock myself in my house with a fridge full of super healthy food, so I devised some strategies and tactics to deal with the real world—whether that be dinner dates, special events, or just nights when you want to grab takeout instead of cooking.

Whatever you do: Do. Not. Stress. **Sugar Free 3** was designed to be doable for everyone. To help you not just survive but thrive, I've detailed how to deal with potentially sticky situations. Bookmark this section and refer to it before your next social gathering, business trip, or takeout run. And if you have a specific situation and need advice, you can get support from the **Sugar Free 3** community. (Go to Openfit.com/**SF3**.com for more details.) The community we've built is one of the secret weapons for successfully navigating the program. We've got you!

And remember, all it takes is a little prep and shifting your mindset. It's just three weeks! I promise, after a few days you'll be hooked on how good you feel—and the knowledge, education, and awareness you acquire will be retained for life.

WHEN YOU'RE EATING OUT

WHEN YOU START paying closer attention to the food that's served at restaurants, parties, and events, you realize something pretty quickly: Sugar reigns supreme.

And I'm not going to downplay this—it's hard as hell to resist partaking when your wingwoman, wife, husband, or co-worker is sucking back chablis or a craft cocktail while you're sipping on a seltzer with lime. Or when you're on a date and want to grill the waiter about the contents of the menu, while your companion contemplates whether you're too high-maintenance to make it to a second date! Or when you're hanging at a football game and getting beer-pressured into tasting the pumpkin ale (your favorite) and foot-long hoagies, and suddenly you're the one passing and intercepting.

Well, none of those occasions—or any others—have the power to derail you when you're armed with the info below. On **Sugar Free 3** you will have plenty to enjoy, and it's adaptable to your lifestyle. Dining out and parties are part of enjoying life, and I'm going to show you how to do that. Armed with a little knowledge and planning, every situation is figure-outable, as my good friend Marie Forleo likes to say.

AT A RESTAURANT

ELIMINATING SUGARY FOODS from your own pantry and filling it with fresh and healthy options is the relatively easy part. Be sure to check Chapter 4 for the whole list of foods to stock up on, and you can find tons of recipes and meal inspiration in this book. Your kitchen is *yours*, your temple, your **SF3** lab, your sugar-free oasis.

But not everyone will be able to prepare every meal in their house for 21 days—I certainly couldn't. And outside your door, it's a whole different world...one filled with chocolate rivers and lollipop trees. Living in New York City, I have pastries staring me down every time I grab a coffee. Pizza or bagel joints dot most blocks, and new gourmet ice cream shops are opening all the time. Wherever you live, I know there are plenty of options tempting you too. Don't fret. Almost every restaurant and menu also has options that are **SF3**-approved and totally delicious, so you won't need to feel like you're on a "diet" or that you're missing out. I have devised these tactics to help.

Investigate First

Along with enabling you to Google your ex and or drop into an Instagram rabbit hole, the Internet is also a great resource for restaurant menus. If you have a business lunch or dinner date, pick the restaurant and look for the menu online and figure out what your options are using the Allowed Food list. If there's an ingredients list, scan it for added sugars using our Sugar AKAs in the back of the book to help. Many major fast food and chain restaurants list their ingredients online.

If the ingredients are not listed, do your best to consider which meals are the least likely to contain added sugars. Make a selection before you even leave the house. This way, when the server asks to take your order, you won't feel rushed or pressured to decide.

Order First

When it comes to choosing not-so-healthy food, your dining companions can sometimes be a bad influence—it's not their fault. Ordering can be contagious—your brain hears your bud order the yummy-sounding fried calamari and then your mouth blurts out, "I'll have that too." Fear not—I have a trick for thwarting temptation. It may seem rude at first, but it works. Be the one to confidently order first. Who knows—perhaps your choice will have a positive domino effect.

Share Smarter Starters

It happens every time I eat with friends: Someone asks, "Should we just get a bunch of appetizers to share?" It's a great way to sample the menu, while cutting down on the cost. But watch out. One minute you're chatting about what film will win Best Picture at the Academy Awards and the next you've nonchalantly grabbed a honey barbecue chicken wing or taken a chomp out of a fried mozzarella stick that's been dunked in sugary marinara sauce. It's second nature...and human nature. Instead, suggest something **Sugar Free 3** approved to share, like a giant salad, seafood tower, or hummus or guacamole and veggies.

Beware of Liquid Sugars

When asked if you "want something to drink?" the safest answers are water, tea, or coffee. If you're ordering the latter two, make sure you ask for them unsweetened: 12 ounces of sweet tea has anywhere from 20 to 30 grams of sugar, putting it right up there with soda (one can of cola has about 39 grams)—and that means tons of empty calories. Or do what I do, order seltzer water with lemon. The bubbles make it feel like I'm drinking something a little more substantial, the lemon lends a bright note, and the crispness pairs well with most meals. (Plus, if you close your eyes real tight, you can pretend it's a vodka soda.)

Ask for Alterations

I've spent enough time waiting tables in my life to know that chefs—or even line cooks—don't love when customers try to tweak their recipes. Well, my position is: I'm a paying customer, so I'm allowed to ask. Many restaurants are more accommodating than they used to be (probably thanks to the rise in gluten- and dairy-free eaters). Politely ask the waiter how they prepare a dish to see if it's breaded or contains any sugar. Request that your proteins be grilled without the glaze or sauce; swap a white burger bun for extra lettuce and tomato, and brown rice for white rice. Get the picture? You can't get what you don't ask for, right?

Change Location

Restaurants now accommodate an array of dietary lifestyles like paleo, gluten-free, and vegan. You can always find some veggies and protein—or a filling salad. So it's unlikely, but over the three weeks you're on **SF3** if you have to eat at a restaurant that has limited foods to eat, like a pizzeria or all-you-can-eat pasta bar, either use your best judgment or suggest an alternate place to eat. And the good news is that many pasta bars now offer zoodles in addition to white pasta.

In my experience, most people are impressed when I tell them I'm eating more healthfully. And when you reveal that you're cutting added sugars, most will say: "I should do that!" So rather than cause aggravation or eye-rolling, it may inspire curiosity, and thus make them more open to choosing a restaurant suited to your meal mission.

What to Eat, Cuisine by Cuisine

OME CUISINES ARE delightfully predictable. Here's what to do if you're eating...

Italian

The Olive Garden may feel like the Garden of Eden, where the tasty stuff is off-limits. (Although apples are allowed in **SF3**.) It starts with the bread basket, filled with refined flours you can't eat right now. After that, you're likely to find white pasta covered in sauces that may contain sugar or wine. If a dish comes with a side of pasta, I simply ask for a side order of vegetables or a salad with vinegar and olive oil—or go for any of these filling dishes:

- ▶ *Antipasto platter*
- ▶ *Carpaccio*
- ▶ *Grilled chicken with pesto*
- ▶ *Grilled or roasted vegetables with olive oil and seasonings*
- ▶ *Caprese salad, aka tomato, basil, and mozzarella*
- ▶ *Grilled chicken with sautéed veggies*
- ▶ *Grilled fish with veggies*
- ▶ *Grilled steak with veggies*

And at the Olive Garden specifically, now they have a Mediterranean menu and gluten-free menu, so you may find:

- ▶ *Zoodles! (zucchini noodles) Ask for garlic and olive oil*
- ▶ *Grilled chicken breast*
- ▶ *Herb-grilled salmon*
- ▶ *Grilled sirloin*

Chinese

I can read your fortune. It says, "No cookie." It also says, "no dumplings" and "no white rice." But you can say "yes" to the following, if you ask the restaurant to keep them NSA:

▶ *Steamed shrimp, tofu, or chicken and broccoli with black bean sauce on the side*

▶ *Stir-fried chicken, beef, or shrimp with vegetables with black bean sauce*

▶ *Steamed veggies*

▶ *Brown rice*

▶ *Egg drop soup*

At P. F. Chang's, go for:

▶ *Edamame*

▶ *Chili-garlic green beans*

▶ *Asian Caesar without wonton croutons*

▶ *Wok stir-fry filet*

▶ *Spinach with garlic*

▶ *Cup of hot and sour soup*

Mexican

Olé? No way. Simply skip the tortilla chips and any flour-wrapped dishes such as burritos and quesadillas and opt for salads, grilled fish, and delicious guacamole, fresh salsa or pico de gallo. Even tacos get a pass if you promise to order corn tortillas.

And you'll find many common dishes that are perfectly fine on this plan, including:

▶ *Grilled shrimp tostada or tacos**

▶ *Fajitas**

▶ *Grilled chicken tostada or tacos**

▶ *Grilled fish tostada or tacos**

▶ *Ceviche*

▶ *Guacamole*

* Corn tortillas only!

At Chipotle, now they have Whole 30 salad bowls, keto bowls, paleo bowls, vegetarian and vegan bowls, all **SF3** approved, or build yourself a salad or brown rice bowl with some or all of the following:

▶ *Protein of your choice*

▶ *Cilantro-lime brown rice*

▶ *Black or pinto beans*

▶ *Cheese*

▶ *Lettuce*

▶ *Fajita vegetables*

▶ *Guacamole*

▶ *Salsa*

"Where's my carne asada?" *You're probably wondering why carne asada—Mexico's delicious spin on steak—isn't listed here. That's because carne asada marinade usually contains orange juice, sugar, or both. Sorry, amigos!*

Japanese

I love Japanese food because there are so many no-fuss and no-sugar-added options:

▶ *Edamame*

▶ *Miso soup*

▶ *Green salad*

▶ *Grilled salmon or chicken with steamed veggies*

▶ *Brown rice*

▶ *Sashimi*

▶ *NaRuto rolls* (rolls wrapped in cucumber without the rice)

Pro Tips: White sushi rice is not allowed for two reasons: it's refined and it's made with sugar to make it sticky. Also, stay away from the pickled ginger. Yes, it's pretty, especially when it's pink, but they use sugar in the pickling process.

American Staples

Most American sit-down chains put sugar in everything—the hamburger buns, the sauces, the glazes, the dressings. Yet it's easy to eat sugar free because most places offer:

▶ *Eggs any style*

▶ *Grilled or steamed seafood*

▶ *Grilled chicken*

▶ *Salad or salad bar (use oil and vinegar as a dressing!)*

▶ *Brown rice*

▶ *Potatoes*

▶ *Avocado*

▶ *Sugar-free condiments like salt, pepper, mustard, lemon, and lime*

At Denny's, enjoy the:

▶ *Three-egg omelet*

▶ *Grilled chicken*

▶ *Grilled haddock*

For more dining out tips visit Openfit.com/SF3.

WHEN YOU'RE ORDERING IN

I LOVE RESTAURANT delivery apps—urbanites practically exist on them, and they are becoming more popular outside of major cities too. As convenient as they are, it's extremely easy to add a bunch of unhealthy fare to your cart—nobody's looking! Simply use the tips and strategies outlined in this book, the Allowed food list, and a little common sense to help. You'll find so many options: salads, burgers (sans bun), sashimi, grilled or roasted chicken. And once you get the hang of this, it will become second nature, and soon you'll wonder how you got by before gaining this knowledge.

What's more, the beauty of takeout or delivered food is you still have access to all the healthy, NSA condiments in your personal pantry, so you can flavor your foods the way you like.

Spice It Yourself

Order your proteins as plain as possible—grilled or steamed is usually best. Then use your own sugar-free sauces or seasonings to spice it up.

Dress It Down

When ordering salads, watch out for other added ingredients, such as candied nuts (one of my biggest pet peeves—why do I need sugar on my salad?), croutons (aka bread), or dried fruit. Then add your own toppings at home, such as toasted slivered almonds, pine nuts, or even dried chickpeas. If you're feeling adventurous, make your own baked croutons from **SF3**-approved sprouted bread.

Dress It Up

Order your salad without dressing and douse it yourself. I'm always exploring new extra virgin olive oils, including flavored ones such as lemon or basil. And there are so many vinegars that I never get tired of salads. Explore all of our delicious NSA recipes at Openfit.com/**SF3**. And see my go-to dressing on page 139.

Take Sides (the right ones)

Just because you'll see "tempura" cauliflower, "honey" glazed carrots, or breaded onion rings doesn't mean all sides are off limits. There are plenty of healthy options out there; remember, the goal is to be satisfied. Most restaurants, even simple diners, have tons of sides that work on the program. Some options: baked or roasted potatoes or sweet potatoes; sautéed, grilled, or steamed broccoli, spinach, asparagus, or green beans; quinoa or brown rice; a green side salad.

WHEN YOU'RE ON THE GO

WHILE TRAVELING, YOU'RE focused on getting from Point A to Point B, not on what to eat. It's tempting to resort to getting a protein bar at a newsstand or a yogurt from an airport kiosk. But the smartest way to take on a travel day is to prepare and plan—you have to get your clothes together, so just carve out a little extra time to get your food together. Eat a healthy and satiating breakfast before you head out the door. Pack yourself some **SF3**-approved snacks you can eat on the run throughout the day (or on the plane). I like to pack some of the following:

- *Plain or dry-roasted nuts*
- *Seed crisps such as Mary's Gone crackers*
- *Hard-boiled eggs (your plane seatmate may not be psyched, but oh, well!)*
- *Sliced apples with NSA peanut butter (nowadays you can often find those convenient individual packets of PB)*
- *Cut-up veggies*

If you can't do that, you can still find **Sugar Free 3**-approved snacks on the go that won't set you back. And as the public gets more health conscious, healthy food is beginning to crop up at airports, which have long-been sugar-free deserts. Some quick picks you're likely to find:

- *Hummus packs*
- *Roasted chickpeas*
- *Almonds*
- *Pistachios*
- *Pumpkin seeds*
- *Popcorn (not kettle corn)*
- *Cheese sticks*
- *Plain yogurt*
- *Fresh fruit*

OTHER SOCIAL SITUATIONS

When You're on a Date

No one wants to be *that* girl or *that* guy—the picky, ask-a-zillion-questions special-request eater. You already feel weird about it...and never more so than on a date.

On **Sugar Free 3**, however, you need to get comfortable with being a little uncomfortable. Here's what you have to remember: You are in control. You are in charge. You are free to be sugar-free for three weeks. And you're not going to apologize for it! As I said earlier, most people will be intrigued when they hear you're on a program to cut added sugars.

Another thing to remember is that every date doesn't have to focus on food. Break away and suggest something else, like going to a movie, concert, or a show, playing Frisbee in the park, or trying a new work-out class. But if you're planning a meal out for your date, follow the dining-out tips. Crib sheet: Research the menu and food items first and have your order ready; pass on alcohol or use this occasion as your mindful indulgence; if your date wants to split an appetizer, suggest vegetables and hummus, grilled shrimp, fresh seafood platter (minus the cocktail sauce), seared tuna, or a salad.

When You're at a Work Party

My favorite *The Office* episodes are the ones featuring the party-planning committee—no matter what they were celebrating, no one had fun. Well, you can. Here's how.

Ask to be a part of the process. With your hand in at the beginning, you can better steer the food and drink choices, including foods that are still delicious crowd pleasers. Steer them toward vegetables and proteins—after all, eating healthy is *in*. Vegetable crudités with healthy dips and spreads, grilled protein skewers, sashimi platters, fresh seafood. Breakfast meetings can offer yogurts, fruit, and hard-boiled eggs, in addition to pastries and bagels. And when designing the dessert spread, strongly suggest that a fruit platter be included so you can partake.

Bring Your Own Dish

If your office party is potluck style, then you're in luck. You know that at least one of the dishes will be **Sugar Free 3**-approved—yours. Be the star with the most tasty and interesting dish. Bonus points if you get the office to make it a "Healthy Potluck" theme. There are a ton of ideas in the book and at Openfit.com/**SF3**. Here are some ideas:

- *A vegetable tray with a variety of hummus spreads (beet, curry, garlic)*
- *Tomato salad marinated in olive oil and fresh herbs*
- *Chopped salad with your favorite homemade dressing*

- *Tex-Mex bowl*
- *Cauliflower rice*
- *Kebobs with an array of spreads*
- *Lettuce cup sliders with our SF3 ketchup*
- *Zucchini pizza boats*
- *Turkey meatballs*
- *Roasted brussels sprouts*
- *Olives*
- *Mediteranean mezze platter*
- *Baked cayenne "fries"*

And if you want to sample some of the yummy options your co-workers brought, just casually ask about the ingredients used for the dishes before diving in.

Make Your Own Spa Water

Spike your water—sparkling or flat—with sliced cucumber, lemon, limes, oranges or strawberries, pineapple or watermelon, even mint. Infusing your water with fruit enhances the taste. Plus it sparks your senses and just makes water more exciting and exotic to drink, so you drink more of it—and drinking more water is always a good thing.

When You're at a Family Gathering

Family gatherings, dinners, and reunions can be some of the hardest situations you'll encounter during the three weeks.

From the sugar-laden foods to the pushy family members who don't understand why you're doing this—they just want you to eat! Maybe your grandmother makes gooey chocolate chip cookies or your uncle is known for his decadent candied yams. You'll have to challenge your own traditions and habits when attending these family functions so you can steer clear of dishes that you know are loaded with sugar. To avoid this added anxiety, try to plan your three weeks away from holidays or family gatherings. If that's unavoidable, stand firm, stay strong, and remember you are in control of you. Hopefully your family will support your admirable efforts. You can always eat beforehand or bring a salad, veggie side, or something you love so you know for sure you'll have something you can enjoy with zero guilt.

When You're at Sporting Events, Concerts, and Movie Theaters

Events and public venues can be tricky, with very few options to eat at the concession stand. Remember you're there for the entertainment, not the food. And fortunately, these events usually only last a couple of hours or so. Ditch temptation by eating before you go, and stay hydrated with a big bottle of water. If you're tailgating, pack a cooler of sugar-free snacks, and if you're really in a jam and need to eat, opt for popcorn, peanuts, or a burger, minus the bun.

When You're Hanging with Your Friends

Your drinking buddies may want to take your new sugar-free lifestyle with a grain of tequila salt, especially when they find out you won't be indulging in adult beverages on girls' or guys' night out. But here's the thing—it's not forever, it's just three short weeks. True friends will support you, and I bet you'll find that you're just as much fun sober as you are after a few cocktails (actually, moreso, since imbibing too much can lead to unnecessary drama). If all else fails, offer to be the designated driver—that usually draws cheers! If it's easier to skip the night out altogether, take a rain check. If you decide to mindfully indulge, enjoy it and get back on track tomorrow.

How to Get Your Mate on Board

Even if they won't join you on the program, they can support your success. Here's how to win them over:

▶ *Ask for their support:* I said it before, but I'll say it again: Explain how important this program is and clearly ask for your love's support. Maybe it should be an expectation, but don't assume your partner knows how much you'd appreciate a little extra backup. They can even help explain it to your mutual friends, if you get tired of repeating (or defending) yourself.

▶ *Get them to hide their stash:* Out of sight, out of mind. Ask your significant other to put sugary foods out of reach and out of your sight line. This will make it easier for you to forget they exist.

▶ *Plan your meals—separately or together:* You two don't have to eat different things during this period, because you'll be eating real food that's delicious and satisfying. (Use the 7-day plans in the book to help in your prep.) I bet your mate will be game to try some of your new recipes. This will save time on meal prep—and money. He or she may be cool with your **Sugar Free 3**-approved bread for a sandwich. You can still enjoy burger night—just skip the bun. And most people will be super satisfied by grilled chicken with our **SF3** marinara. Experimentation—of all kinds—keeps relationships interesting.

CHAPTER

HOW TO CRUSH A CRAVING

Lusting for a Sweet Fix?
Strategies for Resisting Sugar's Seductive Pull

"I've been hangry all day."
"My sweet tooth booty called me late last night."
"I'm feeling snacky after dinner."
"I need a piece of chocolate!"

COMMENTS LIKE THESE came during week one from the very first people to try **Sugar Free 3**. Listening to them, I realized how important support is during the early stages of the program—the struggle is real, and I can totally relate! On my day six, I stepped off an elevator at an event and was greeted by the prettiest tray of rosé champagne. I turned to my friend and said, rather dramatically, "This is killing me." Resisting that time did kinda hurt.

To help prevent you from caving in moments like that, I made this program as doable as possible by providing as much support and as many tools as I could. Sugar cravings can be strong—sweet foods are tempting us at every turn, and for many of us, consuming those foods is longtime habit that we associate with comfort or celebration. Bottom line, cutting added sugars isn't easy! But **Sugar Free 3** can be. My advice for bolstering your willpower and silencing sugar's obnoxious come-ons will propel you on this healthy journey.

SILENCE THE CALL

SOMETIMES SUGAR WHISPERS at you from the grocery store aisle; other times it screams at you from the freezer. Regardless, you can learn to silence those calls. First, it helps to know what a craving is. Webster's Dictionary defines it as "an intense, urgent, or abnormal desire or longing." Synonyms include: yearning, hankering, desire, wish, want, lust. Sounds about right when it comes to describing how I feel about chocolate!

One of the biggest takeaways I got during my three weeks: Just because you're having a "craving" or "want" something sweet doesn't mean you have to eat sugar—or even pop a sugar replacement, such as a piece of fruit—on impulse. Fortify your resistance by understanding what's really going on. Do you...

> *...want chocolate or just something sweet?*
> *...feel physical hunger and is your stomach growling?*
> *...have a headache?*

Then, once answered:

◆ Drink a glass of water.

◆ Take a breather—5 deep breaths—or wait a few minutes.

◆ Try to do something physical such as taking a short walk.

◆ Eat something if you're truly hungry. Just make sure that something satiates you. When a craving hit, many in our test group would grab fruit (seemingly, the most obvious fix). But fruit alone may not quell the craving—especially if it isn't necessarily for something sweet. Your best bet for stamping out a craving—of any kind—may be to have a snack that also includes protein or a healthy fat.

My Snack Hacks

SWEET *A few things to satisfy your screaming sweet tooth.*

▶ Fruit with almond butter

▶ Fruit with a handful of nuts

▶ Fruit with plain Greek yogurt

▶ Openfit Plant-Based Protein Shake

▶ Recipes
  • *Cherries and Ricotta with Almonds*
  • *Baked Cinnamon Apple*

▶ An herbal tea that has a sweet note such as vanilla

SALTY *Treats such as barbecue chips can have added sugars. Try these instead.*

▶ Guac and cucumber "chips"

▶ Veggies and hummus (when I want crunch)

▶ **SF3**-approved crackers and hummus

▶ Biltong or some other kind of jerky (turkey, salmon) when I want something savory

▶ Handful of nuts or seeds. I go for pistachios in the shell— they take longer to eat

▶ Hard-boiled egg

*Be sure to check out my snack list and recipes in Chapter 5 of the book and more recipes at Openfit.com/**SF3**.*

Expert Snack Hacks

"I like to snack on raw or dry roasted nuts, fresh fruit and vegetables, and a sugar-free type of African beef jerky called biltong," says Max Lugavere, author of *Genius Foods*. "I often pack these items in my bag when I'm on the go."

"I'll have an apple and peanut butter," says nutritionist Keri Glassman. "Or mash up an avocado and dip veggies into it. For some kind of crunch, I like some gluten-free crackers or grain-free tortilla chips."

Nighttime Cravings

We all know those after-dinner times when you're just feeling "noshy" or want that post-meal sweet indulgence. Here are some tactics that worked for our test group:

◆ Drink water

◆ Brush your teeth; who wants to taint a fresh mouth and fresh breath?

◆ Do yoga or meditate

◆ Meal prep or search for **SF3** recipes

◆ Last resort, use your Mindful Indulgence

Are You Hungry or Just Thirsty?

Sometimes—a lot of times, actually—thirst can be sneaky, masquerading as hunger. The cues are similar: you might get a headache, feel lethargic, your stomach may rumble, or you might have difficulty concentrating if you're thirsty or hungry. My rule of thumb: Drink half your weight in ounces every day. So if you weigh 150 pounds, drink 75 ounces of water. You might find your hunger pangs decrease too. If you're experiencing headaches, which is totally expected the first 5 days, down more H2O! Keri shared these awesome tips with me:

GET A NEW WATER BOTTLE

"Since some of your meals will not be eaten at home, invest in a BPA-free, refillable water bottle that you can carry with you—everywhere. I always recommend snagging one that holds 32 ounces, so you just have to remember to fill it twice in one day, and *boom*! 64 ounces down the hatch."

SAVOR AN HERBAL TEA

"If you're sipping it, it gets you through the moment, and some can taste sweet."

GO FOR BUBBLES

"Replace your glass of water at one meal today with a tall glass of seltzer water. You don't need the bubbles from champagne to feel a little festive, and who says champagne glasses are only for champagne? Here's permission to get fancy sans alcohol."

ADD BASIC FLAVOR

"Boost your water with the juice of a lemon wedge or slice up your favorite fruit. Not only will this give your water a little extra flavor (making you want to drink more), the added antioxidants can give you a little extra perk."

TRY A SPICY WATER

"Kickstart your day by adding a pinch or two of cayenne pepper to your water. The capsaicin in the cayenne gives your metabolism a marginal boost. Plus, it gives you that little jolt to make sure you're really paying attention to your hydration."

STOP A CRAVING BEFORE IT STARTS

Tactics you can use over the three weeks to sidestep a lapse

BEWARE OF SUGAR PUSHERS

ONE OF THE epiphanies you are bound to have on this sugar-busting quest is that sugary foods are lurking everywhere—at the juice bar, in the ballpark, even your kids' doctor's office! Another realization: While most people are going to support your get-healthy mission, there will be a few who try to derail your efforts. I call them the sugar pushers. They are people who tend to make you feel bad when you don't partake. At a birthday or holiday dinner you might notice your mom is trying to persuade you to eat dessert, or your friends are eye-rolling because you turned down a cocktail. Even your spouse (your in-home support system!) can morph into a sugar pusher because he or she wants to hit that all-you-can-eat pasta joint. A few tips: I highly recommend that you not only tell your friends, family, co-workers, and significant other that you are embarking on **Sugar Free 3**, you need to go the extra step of actively asking them for their encouragement and cooperation. If they still try to lure you to eat foods that are not **SF3**-approved, stay strong and know this: It's not about you, it's about them. It's about them not feeling fantastic about their own choices and not wanting to be left behind. Stick to the plan, and after a few failed attempts, they will likely stop trying to lead you astray. Better yet, your compliance could inspire them to make some positive changes of their own.

Start a Movement

▶ *Get Your Buds on Board.* If Friday nights were usually reserved for chicken wings and beer, propose a new tradition these next three weeks. You could turn wing night into a board game night at your place, where you're in charge of the menu—and the "drinks."

▶ *Find New Friends.* It may be time to open yourself up to the possibility of hanging out with new friends who are also attempting to live a healthier lifestyle. Spending time with other people who are kicking the sugar habit can make it easier for you to enjoy your free time without temptation. You can eat healthy meals together, join in on activities that don't center around food or drink, share meal ideas, confide in each other about the struggles of your lifestyle change, and compare motivational strategies. You can meet people like this in the **Sugar Free 3** online community.

▶ *Take a Detour.* If you used to take a specific route to work so you could stop by a bakery for a donut and coffee, it's time to switch up your daily commute. You may be strong enough to avoid that bakery every day, but why tempt fate?

AUDIT YOUR EATING

OMETIMES THE SOURCE of cravings can be uncovered if you take a closer look at what you're eating and when. Factors to address include:

◆ *Achieving Balance.* Make sure your meals are balanced (protein, veggies and/or other healthy carbs, and healthy fats) from the Totally Allowed list and the Allowed in Moderation list at every meal.

◆ *Having a Snack Strategy.* If you're having afternoon cravings, work an afternoon snack into your routine.

◆ ***Pacing Your Meals Properly.*** This may require some work, but it's important to plan the eating cadence ahead of time. This can help prevent you from getting too hungry during the day, which leads to voracious munching and overeating.

◆ ***Adjusting Your Mealtimes.*** On **Sugar Free 3**, I recommend *what* to eat for your three meals and one or two snacks. But I don't tell you *when* to eat them. I personally eat breakfast in the morning, lunch at lunchtime, etc. If you feel tired or cravings are hitting, identify times of the day. For example, after a few days of observation, you might conclude that around 3 p.m. every day, your energy is depleted, you crave sugar, and you feel extremely hungry. This might be a signal to add a protein-filled snack at this time of day to power through— maybe a shake or two hard-boiled eggs, or a handful of nuts, or have some apple slices with peanut butter. Not only will this make you feel better instantly, it also sets you up for a better evening, and fewer cravings around bedtime.

◆ ***Spicing Things Up.*** It's possible to get stuck in an eating rut on **Sugar Free 3**, eating the same simple meals every day because you know they're "safe." But as they say, variety is the spice of life—and spice is a savior when you're swapping out sugar. Some of the best unique flavors are derived from easily accessible spices that don't contain any added sugar. You'll find a few in Chapter 5.

◆ ***Identifying Your Faves.*** If you're eating a salad with grilled chicken and it's totally unsatisfying, you're going to crave a sweet more in the afternoon as opposed to if you enjoyed a healthy taco salad that might be really satisfying. Work harder to figure out what you love so you're satisfied in general—so you don't feel deprived. I try to keep it simple and pick two go-to breakfasts, two go-to lunches, and two go-to dinners each week so I can stay consistent.

◆ ***Getting Curious.*** Explore our recipes, exchange ideas in our online community, try some new fruits and vegetables you've never even heard of, or combine different ingredients to create new dishes. By switching up what you're eating from day to day, you might find a new delicious dish that gets you excited about Tuesday night's dinner. Hey, it could happen!

How Sleep Is Connected to Shedding Pounds

While many people report better, longer, and sounder sleep, not everyone has an easy time getting a good night's slumber. Sleep is critical, and sometimes not getting enough leaves us hungry and "craving" foods we ordinarily wouldn't crave. Studies recommend getting 6–8 hours, no more, no less. If you're not getting enough sleep, be aware that you may find yourself hankering for more carb-filled foods. My suggestions for helping get a good night's sleep include regular exercise, cutting off caffeine consumption by 3 p.m., scenting your room with sleep-inducing scents such as lavender, taking a hot bath or shower (when your body cools, it is lulled to sleep—it's biology), observing an electronic sunset, where you stop using digital devices a few hours before bed, and wearing a silky sleep mask to block out stray light.

TREAT YOURSELF AFTER REACHING MILESTONES

YOU WILL BE constantly rewarded for doing **Sugar Free 3**—with weight loss, higher energy levels, better skin, and sounder sleep. But setting smaller goals throughout the process and celebrating yourself when you reach them will also keep you on track.

Decide which milestones you want to reward yourself for before starting the program. Maybe it's after completing the first week without eating any added sugars. Maybe it's after a win like going to your favorite restaurant—and saying no to the ribs drenched in sugary barbecue sauce. Some of the things I like to treat myself with.

• *Mani/pedi with foot massage*

- *Workout outfit*
- *New kitchen gadget*
- *Midday movie*

You could also implement smaller, more immediate rewards. A recent study proved they boost motivation. "The idea that immediate rewards could increase intrinsic motivation sounds counterintuitive, as people often think about rewards as undermining interest in a task," said Cornell researcher Kaitlin Woolley, who, with Ayelet Fishbach, published research in the *Journal of Personality and Social Psychology*. "But for activities like work, where people are already getting paid, immediate rewards can actually increase intrinsic motivation, compared with delayed or no rewards." Your immediate reward could also be a quiet hour alone watching TV, a quick nap, or luxuriating with a book in a bath.

Your reward could also be—wait for it—the Mindful Indulgence you are allowed on the **SF3** program! One early tester said her peanut butter cup never tasted as sweet as it did after she ate it as a reward for finishing week one. On the other hand, many people felt so good that they didn't even want to indulge. And that's awesome too!

BREAK A SWEAT

WHEN PEOPLE START this program they often ask if they can exercise, thinking it's a detox or a cleanse that will leave them too lethargic to get their butts moving and break a sweat. The truth is, you'll probably have more energy when you do **Sugar Free 3**—I know I did. I was astounded, actually, because I consider myself a pretty energetic person to begin with. But this plan supplied a surplus.

So yes, you can (and are encouraged to) exercise on this plan, with a few caveats. A diet change can affect your body and how it functions, so if you're a big exerciser, your previous routine may feel a little more difficult at first as your body adjusts. Stick with it and do what you can. You will adapt. If you've been eating a lot of sugar prior to starting you may find yourself tired the first few days, and even experience headaches. That is totally normal and expected and is your body's way of letting go of the sugar crutch and getting used to the healthy foods you're now providing it with. Take a few more days of rest, then get back to it! Your energy levels should rebound—and possibly even increase—quickly, so now might be an awesome time to add exercise to your regime.

If you're looking for new options, sign up for Openfit at Openfit. com/**SF3**. Not only can you access my video-based companion to this program, but you'll find all kinds of on-demand and live workouts from cardio to barre to yoga. Plus, brand-new 15-minute movement workouts from my friend Lauren Roxburgh, who is a fitness and alignment expert. (Her nickname is "The Body Whisperer.") The workouts are specifically designed to support you on your **Sugar Free 3** path. "You'll roll away the tension and boost circulation," says Lauren. "And you'll feel lighter and fully relaxed. I call it movement medicine."

Additionally, if your energy levels have boosted to epic proportions, you can add new activities to your leisure time, such as walking, hiking, or biking. These positive habits can distract you from the tough changes you're making to your diet—and keep your hands out of the cookie jar.

KEEP TRACK

W HETHER IT'S ON the Openfit app or writing in a journal or just keeping notes on your phone, food tracking is proven to help people reach their goals. According to a study funded by the National Heart, Lung and Blood Institute at the National Institutes of Health, diet participants who kept a daily food journal were twice as likely to lose weight as dieters who didn't keep any food records at all. While your **Sugar Free 3** goal may not be weight loss, the simple act of writing down what you're eating forces you to confront your daily habits and ensure added sugars aren't sneaking into your diet.

You can track what you're eating, how you're handling cravings, and other feelings and achievements. Our test group tracked:

- *What they ate and drank (including water intake)*
- *When they ate and drank*
- *Any Mindful Indulgences*
- *When cravings reared their ugly heads*
- *How they felt physically and mentally*
- *If they exercised*
- *"Aha" moments or epiphanies and also struggles*

If you're feeling fab and energized, jot it down. If you have a headache, a craving, or you're just having a tough time, write that down too. This way, you can see your daily emotional highs and lows and you can identify patterns. By connecting your feelings to the foods you're eating, you can begin to understand which foods make you feel good and which foods are making it hard to stick to your lifestyle change.

SURPRISING SECRET WEAPONS

These wellness-driven, outside-the-box ideas
can help give you the edge you need

EATING MINDFULLY

THE BASICS OF mindful eating are pretty simple: You savor your food as you eat it by engaging all of your senses, and you eat it slowly. This leads to a more considered approach to eating, and thus more responsible choices. In fact, mindful eating starts before you eat. It's about deciding: Do I really want this? What is my body—not my mind—telling me? With practice and some tricks of the mindfulness trade, like the tips I previewed in one of my earlier books *20 Pounds Younger*, you can learn to do it effectively and discover mindful eating is not about deprivation, it's about choice. Some pointers:

Consider Your Choice

If you can condition yourself to pause and consider your food choice before you commit your tongue, you have learned a great secret of mindful eating. German researchers sorted the reasons we eat into 15 core motives.

Check 'em out; you'll recognize many of your own drivers for diving in that have nothing to do with being hungry. Getting to know them is one key to mastering mindful eating.

- *Liking:* I eat this food because it tastes good.

- *Habit:* This is something I'm accustomed to eating regularly.

- *Need and hunger:* I am hungry or need an energy boost.

◆ *Health:* I'm trying to maintain a balanced diet or stay in shape, and this food achieves that goal.

◆ *Convenience:* This food is quick or easy to prepare, convenient, or readily available.

◆ *Pleasure:* I want to indulge or reward myself. This food puts me in a good mood.

◆ *Tradition:* My family always eats this food on this holiday. I always snack on this food during this activity.

◆ *Natural concerns:* This food is organic, fair trade, environmentally friendly, or natural.

◆ *Sociability:* It's pleasant to eat with others. Eating makes social gatherings more enjoyable or comfortable.

◆ *Price:* This item is inexpensive, on sale, free, or I've already purchased it.

◆ *Visual appeal:* The package is appealing, the food is nicely presented.

◆ *Weight control:* This food is low in fat or calories, and I'm trying to lose weight.

◆ *Emotional regulation:* I'm sad, frustrated, lonely, bored, or stressed, and this food cheers me up.

◆ *Social norms:* It would be impolite not to eat this—I wouldn't want to disappoint.

◆ *Social image:* This food is trendy right now and reinforces the image I want to portray.

Snack Up

Snacks keep hunger at bay so you don't run to the vending machine at work or grab a Friday doughnut at the office. If you have them handy every day, you won't be tempted by sugar-filled or calorie-dense packaged foods. Making your own at the beginning of the week helps you be proactive about mindful eating and gives you the goods for healthier snacking.

Pretend You're a Food Critic

Your job isn't just to scarf down the food on your plate—you have to take note of the presentation, the nuances of every flavor, and how satisfying each item is. "When you bite into a grape, all of these juices come out—and there are sensations you'd totally miss if you just stuffed a handful of grapes into your mouth," says Katie Rickel, PhD, a clinical psychologist and weight-loss expert who works at a weight-management facility in Durham, North Carolina. "Try to follow the first bite down your esophagus and into your belly, and take a moment to notice whether you feel one grape more energetic." In mindful eating workshops, people first practice this with just three or four raisins. "That really brings people's attention down to their sensory experience," says Jennifer Daubenmier, PhD, an assistant professor at the Osher Center for Integrative Medicine at the University of California—San Francisco. "They really notice the texture, the smell, and the thoughts that come up."

Observe Your Inner Experience

You can drag out your meal for two hours, but all of that extra time doesn't mean a thing if you aren't paying attention to what's happening inside your body and mind. To truly be mindful, you need to take note of every sensation and urge: How do I know when I'm hungry? What sensations do I experience? What does it feel like when I'm emotionally, but not physically, hungry? How do I know when I'm full?

Your Mindful Indulgence. *If these craving crushers aren't doing the trick and you've got to "break glass in case of emergency," enjoy your once-a-week Mindful Indulgence. It's the perfect opportunity to practice mindful eating, and it's built into the plan for exactly that reason.*

Use Aromatherapy to Outsmart Cravings

ALOT OF PEOPLE have a therapist. I have an *aroma*therapist. Her name is Michelle Gagnon, and she actually calls herself a "bio alchemist," which may be the coolest job title ever. I met her working with The Well, a member-based wellness club in New York City. Michelle travels the world and works, in her words, "exclusively with wildcrafted/organic botanical ingredients and essential oils sourced from farms and artisan distilleries around the world." Her expert curation of these aromatic materials create "a luxurious botanical olfaction experience evoking healing benefits while allowing us to live in harmony with nature and our environment."

Not to mention, they smell damn good.

When I told Michelle I was doing this book, she had some terrific insights about how aromatherapy could help you crush cravings on **Sugar Free 3**, and I wanted to share my interview with her so that you could benefit from her impressive wisdom.

Is it true that sense of smell and appetite are intertwined?

Absolutely. Our sense of smell is the most primordial of our senses and has a great impact on our sense of taste. In fact 80 to 90 percent of what we think we are tasting we are actually smelling. If you have ever walked by a kitchen where the aroma of a freshly cooked meal has made you salivate or triggered hunger, then you have experienced the power of scent affecting your appetite. We process odor in the same part of the brain as memory and emotion, linked to past and personal experiences.

You're making me think of those cinnamon bun stands in the mall. Every time I walk by one, I'm reminded of going to the mall as a kid, and I suddenly crave a 1,000-calorie blob of dough.

Right. If you enjoy a freshly baked pastry in the morning, the odor emanating from the bakery's door will stimulate your appetite, just as vanilla essential oil may as well. If you enjoy eating meat, the aroma of slowly roasted meat may stimulate your appetite, whereas if you are a vegetarian it may suppress it. Although scent is a personal journey, there are a few essential oils that we can access to help combat cravings, and promote homeostasis within the body. The beautiful thing about working with essential oils is that they are holistic in and of themselves, and work on our holistic well-being, affecting the physical, emotional, and spiritual body.

Which scents help with feeling less hungry?

Citrus essential oils, such as grapefruit, lemon, orange, and bergamot can assist in curbing the appetite, especially grapefruit with its high content of d-limonene. D-limonene is a terpene found in the peel of citrus fruits, where its essential oil is stored, and is a potent antioxidant with anti-inflammatory properties. It is also a great aid in curbing cravings and appetite.

Other chemical constituents found in citrus essential oils offer uplifting properties that can lift the spirit and mood and promote energy. A few others I recommend:

- ▶ Believe it or not, cinnamon bark essential oil can also help curb sweet cravings, while making you feel satisfied and warm as well.
- ▶ Essential oils such as anise, basil, and peppermint can actually stimulate the appetite, supporting healthy digestion and metabolism.
- ▶ I work with peppermint essential oil often as a digestive, and find it has somewhat adaptogenic properties.

By adaptogenic, you mean it helps counteract stress?

Exactly. I have experienced peppermint to be relaxing and energizing, depending on what the body needs. It gives the sensation a meal is finished and can curb the craving for something sweet afterwards. An infusion of herbal peppermint tea can also provide this feeling.

What scents might help anyone having a hard time getting through these three weeks?

Geranium and lavender can provide great support on **Sugar Free 3**, as they can help ease and calm the mind and help support the challenges that may arise physically and emotionally. They are great at promoting balance and homeostasis as well as a good night's sleep.

How should we use these oils? Diffuse them? Pour in the tub?

I suggest working with essential oils via topical application (with caution) and via inhalation. A simple inhale of essential oil triggers their effects. When we smell, we smell with our brains. The odor molecules come into direct contact with the brain, where scent receptors receive, interpret, and transmit the messages these chemical signals offer to various parts of the body. It happens so fast that before we are aware we have smelled something our brain and body have already reacted to it.

Alternatively you can apply a couple drops of essential oil to a cotton ball to keep in your pocket and inhale throughout the day or as cravings arise, or add a few drops to a diffuser. I suggest diffusing grapefruit and lemon during the day and a combination of lavender and orange in the diffuser at night, for a comforting night's sleep.

For a refreshing mist you can mix 10–15 drops of essential oil in 1 ounce of distilled water (which can be found at most grocery stores) and mist onto your skin throughout the day, taking a moment for a long, long inhale. (Try any of the essential oils I've mentioned or a combination of two.) Working with these materials with intention also provides the opportunity to reflect and reinforce your manifestation.

Sometimes I rub essential oils into my temple—especially when I have a headache. I use peppermint for that.

Our skin is our largest organ and things we apply to it get absorbed by our bodies and pass through our bloodstream. Applying essential oils topically is a beautiful way to receive their beneficial properties for the skin and the body as a whole.

Apply 15 drops of essential oil to 1 oz. of your moisturizer or into a carrier oil such as jojoba, avocado, or apricot kernel oil and massage onto clean, damp skin. Citrus essential oils have a mild exfoliating effect on the skin so be cautious—there are photo compounds in citrus essential oils that can cause photosensitivity to the skin when applied and exposed to direct sunlight.

Geranium balances not only the inner workings of the body but the skin as well, and is great for all skin types.

START MEDITATING

MANY YEARS BACK, I got trained in Transcendental Meditation (TM) because that practice—which entails doing 20 minutes of a mantra-based meditation in the morning and then again later in the day—has so many amazing health benefits. But you don't have to be an experienced meditator to reap the benefits. A little mindfulness can go a long way when it comes to making yourself feel amazing. According to a review of research published in the journal *JAMA Internal Medicine*, meditation and mindfulness can help reduce stress, anxiety, and even physical pain—all in as little as 10 minutes a day. Even though I fall off my practice now and then, I tried to adhere to it during **Sugar Free 3** because it really helps. It's a secret weapon against cravings—but a really peaceful one. Below are a few of the reasons I love meditating, and the research behind why it works.

It Helps Reduce Anxiety

Truly. And biologically. There is evidence to suggest that meditation does, in fact, modify our neurological functions in a way that helps combat the imagined fears that characterize an anxiety attack.

As a journalist, even one steeped in wellness, I was skeptical of meditation at first. I looked for "proof" and found that researchers at Massachusetts General Hospital and Harvard Medical School asked 42 participants to complete an eight-week yoga and meditation course designed to reduce stress. They also asked a control group of 25 participants to complete an eight-week course in which they engaged in light aerobic exercise and were taught about the impact of stress. MRI brain scans showed that those who completed the yoga and meditation course showed changes in the hippocampus—the area of the brain associated with learning and emotions—in ways that helped mitigate their feelings of unreal or imaginary threat.

It Energizes You

In today's culture of information overload, we all need to quiet our thoughts and be more present. Meditation helps center you. It also provides a natural energy boost. "I meditate once every morning," says movement and mindfulness teacher Lauren Roxburgh, "and find it gives me a renewed strength to face each day stronger."

It Helps You Control Your Thoughts—and Cravings

Put simply, mindful meditation simply enables us to better monitor our thoughts and, in doing so, regulate our emotional responses to them. And thus we reach for the gummy bears less often. "Imagine that instead of believing that you are your thoughts, you see yourself as an external observer of them," says Omri Kleinberger, the CEO and founder of the corporate meditation and yoga company Ometa in New York City. "During an anxious episode"—or, say, a sugar craving—"it is common for people to think things like, 'Everything is falling apart and I have no control over it.' Every time you have that thought, it reinforces the stress-inducing emotions associated with it. In meditation, you learn to become mindfully more aware of your thoughts, so that when you experience a negative thought such as that, you can recognize it as being nothing more than just a thought, and let it go."

Guided Visualizations to Quiet Cravings

*To strengthen your resolve, wellness educator Lauren Roxburgh developed short audio visualizations specifically for **Sugar Free 3**, available on the Openfit app. In them, "we do a body scan in the beginning where we identify discomfort. Then I'll guide you through mindful breathing and motivational thought creation, which is very grounding," says Lauren. "Afterwards, you'll feel a sense of calmness that will help you make better choices and resist temptation. Use these visualizations when you want to destress, increase energy, or are feeling vulnerable. It can be two minutes, 10 minutes—or however long you like."*

GIVE YOURSELF A BREAK

No ONE IS perfect, and while **Sugar Free 3** encourages you to cut out added sugars from your diet for the full three weeks, you may have a slip-up or two. If you do have a bite of ice cream or a gulp of soda, don't freak out and fall into a guilt spiral. The worst thing you can do after a screw-up is to give up or beat yourself up.

Turning a mistake into a full-on sugar-binge sesh will undo all the hard work you've already done. It'll also spike your blood sugar levels and lead to a sugar crash later, which can amplify the guilt and disappointment you might feel about cheating. (You might also make innocent mistakes. "I ordered an In-n-Out burger and asked them to remove the special sauce," reported one early tester, "but I realized after the first bite, they left it on." Rather than keep eating it, he sent it back, although it wouldn't have been the end of the world if he kept eating it.)

If you lose focus, it's important to identify what triggered you. Maybe you had a confrontation with your boss at work that day, got into a fight with your spouse, or simply put yourself in a situation that was too tempting, such as Sunday brunch with your friends. On day two Lynn K. had a rough day teaching, and "would normally jump up to get an ice cream or a donut—something for comfort—but was so excited I was on this sugar-free movement, have the support of the community, and I know I'll get more benefits in the long run."

I love that she was able to identify her trigger (and that she didn't grab that donut—go Lynn!). Address the root cause and you'll be able to cope with your stress in a healthier way.

"Take every meal one step at a time," advises Keri Glassman, the registered dietitian. "Don't think of three weeks. That's overwhelming. Instead, think of the next meal. The next craving. If you go day by day, it's going to be easier."

THE KEEP IT GOING PLANS

Maintenance Ideas for Day 22 and Beyond!

T'S DAY 22. Now what? Can you go out and eat pizza and ice cream? Sure, but do you *really* want to do that? And will you feel good about that tomorrow? My hope is that you're feeling great and enjoying the taste of real, wholesome food like veggies, proteins, and fresh fruit. And maybe your taste buds have adjusted so a sweet potato or a ripe strawberry are the yummy, delicious treats they should be. So why wouldn't you want to keep eating this way? I know I do.

I was thrilled when Michele D., an Openfit employee and one of the first people to test the program, told me she was going to go beyond the 21 days, saying, "Once you're aware of all the added sugars hidden in our processed food, you can't unsee that!" So true!

But we all have different lifestyles and goals, and you need to find a path that's flexible and adaptable so you can stick with it. That's why I created three ways—based on three different personality types—for you to continue, so no matter where you are, how active you plan to be, or how closely you're willing to follow the core principles, you can still feel the benefits of a sugar-free (or sugar-free-ish) life. And no matter your type, you'll want to follow these 6 steps for maintenance success:

◆ *Continue to use the Allowed/Not Allowed lists as your guide for meal planning.* Ground your meals with a balance of healthy proteins and a colorful spectrum of vegetables, grains, fruit, and healthy fats—and continue to keep added sugars, refined carbs, and artificial sweeteners out of your shopping cart.

◆ *Remember, no calorie counting and no portion control!* Some people prefer to do it "by the numbers," but many of us really don't want to deal with all the math that comes from counting calories. Personally, I'm not a calorie counter, but the beauty of the program is that when you eat a balance of the foods in the Allowed category and avoid those that are Not Allowed you don't have to get hung up on details. Yes, you still need to eat things like cheese in moderation, but I don't consider that portion control or calorie counting as much as I consider it common sense.

◆ *Track what you eat.* Inevitably, higher calorie foods from the Allowed in Moderation category and even the Not Allowed list may creep back in. We've all experienced one cookie turning into five. That's why I always recommend that people make note of what they eat, whether that's a mental note, a food journal, or an online meal tracker. It will help you gain better awareness and be more mindful of your food choices, and it only takes a few minutes a day.

◆ *Read labels.* Keep reading those Nutrition Facts and ingredient lists— remember sugar hides out in so many packaged foods, condiments, even so-called "healthy" foods. For example, one serving of low-fat yogurt from popular brands can pack 15 or 16 grams of added sugar, making it closer to an indulgence than a virtuous snack.

◆ *Exercise as much as—or more than!—usual.* As you know, you're not required to exercise during **Sugar Free 3**. The focus was mostly on diet, because, as they say, 80 percent of abs are built in the kitchen. Personally, I exercise regularly and I'm always going to advocate that regular physical activity be part of a healthy lifestyle—besides, you need to expend some of the bonus energy you get from eating less sugar. A good place to kick-start being more active is at Openfit.com, where there are hundreds of workouts and Openfit Live trainer-led small group classes. Of course, if you have any current health issues, it's important to talk with your doctor about starting an exercise program.

◆ *Plan and prep.* If at all possible, plan your week or even just three days at a time. Whether that means deciding where and what you're eating out, going grocery shopping, or experimenting with recipes and meal prep, it doesn't have to be complicated. As you've probably seen, you can make a lot of different meals with a few basic ingredients from the Allowed/Not Allowed list.

OK, so those are the foundational basics. Now, which personality type are you?

THE CONVERT

I T'S SAID THAT all good things must come to an end, to which I reply, "Not true!" If you're loving your new sugar-free life and want to continue feeling great and reaping all the health benefits—or if you still have weight you want to lose—just continue following the program and the maintenence tips.

◆ *One Mindful Indulgence a week.* Continue as you have for the past three weeks, choose mindfully, always enjoy it, and realize that a few bites is usually all you need to be satisfied.

THE WELL-INTENTIONED

I'D PROBABLY PUT myself in this category. I can manage to be a fairly clean eater most of the time, but I want the freedom to enjoy wine with dinner a few times a week—for starters. If you can relate, then in your maintenance phase, follow the 6 tips, with this one adjustment:

♦ *Allow Yourself a Mindful Indulgence 2–3 times a week.* Whether it's a cocktail, chocolate, white-rice sushi, a bagel—or whatever your favorite food is from the Not Allowed list—choose your treats mindfully. Enjoy them! Remember that a few bites (or sips) is usually all you need to be satisfied. "I definitely want to continue following many of the healthy habits from this program. It's worth it, since it makes me feel so good!" says Hannah R., an Openfit employee. "And I want to stay as mindful of my 'indulgences' as possible. When I start thinking of them as treats, they become way more satisfying!"

THE REALIST

YOU'RE SWAMPED WITH professional and personal demands, which may mean eating out most days, or you like to have a glass of wine at dinner, or you're a parent and it's a little harder to avoid the foods on the Not Allowed list. And let's be honest, if you had a glass of wine at dinner and a slice of pizza, that isn't so bad. If you can relate, then you're a realist, and this one's for you. Follow my 6 tips, with one small change:

♦ *Enjoy 1–2 Mindful Indulgences a day.* It's totally fine, as long as you cut out all the other sugar you were eating. You'll still get results.

"I will continue with **Sugar Free 3**," says Jonathan R. from our test group, "but have made a few tweaks that fit my life. For example, I like a small bowl of pasta, or a little ice cream after dinner, I'm totally OK with that. One to two indulgences a day is great and so much less sugar than I used to eat. I am so much healthier now and so much more knowledgeable, and I can live this way forever."

Meal Prep in Four Easy Steps

MEAL PREP MAY seem a little bit daunting at first, but think about it: By spending a couple of hours on, say, Sunday to plan your meals for the week and doing some cooking, you'll be able to come home after running late with a meeting or kids' soccer practice to a ready-to-heat-and-eat meal. You can spend the extra time you gain from the advance work relaxing or hanging out with the fam (imagine).

▶ *Get prepared.* Buy reusable containers (glass ones are the most sustainable) that you can use to store prepped meals in the fridge or take with you to work. There are affordable options available online.

▶ *Keep it simple to start.* Aim for no-fuss combinations like salmon and greens for lunch, or chicken, brown rice, and broccoli for dinner.

▶ *Make a list.* Stock up on versatile basics such as frozen proteins and vegetables. Order in advance from a grocery delivery service to save additional time.

▶ *Be inspired.* Meal prep is trending—now and always. So there is no shortage of healthy, delicious ideas online. You can check out dozens of meal prep ideas and tips at Openfit.com.

How to Drink Responsibly

I'm always asked about drinking wine and other alcohol on this program. And while it's not allowed for three weeks, I wanted to address the subject. Here are my tips:

If you're used to consuming alcohol daily, first and foremost drink in moderation: 1–2 standard drinks.
I don't recommend it, but if you have a big night out where you plan to have multiple drinks, plan for it using these four tips:

▶ *Minimize the sugar during the day.* Remember to stick with the foods on the Allowed list and avoid the Not Allowed list.

▶ *Don't binge drink.* Honestly, most of us have had one too many at some point in our lives. It happens. But setting out for the evening with the intention of getting loaded is never a good idea. With this in mind, pace yourself. According to the Centers for Disease Control, binge drinking is when a man consumes 5 or more drinks or a woman consumes 4 or more drinks in about 2 hours. Try to stay below those limits.

▶ *Avoid the sugary mixers!* Flavored soda, juice, and tonic add additional sugar-laden calories that you're probably not enjoying all that much anyway. Stick to drinking alcohol neat, on the rocks, or mixed with plain, calorie-free club soda. It's best to avoid diet soda as a mixer too; artificial sweeteners may increase appetite and will just make you more snacky (yes, I made that word up, but you get it, right?).

▶ *Forgive yourself if you mess up.* I'm not giving you permission to eff up, but if your night out turns into a late-night pizza and ice cream binge, don't go into a guilt-fueled tailspin. The next day, drink more water and eat a healthy breakfast. Onward!

FINAL WORDS

S O NOW THAT you've identified your personality, you'll see how maintaining **Sugar Free 3** can be very simple. Just make sure your Mindful Indulgences are just that—mindful. Whatever you choose as your treat, slow down and savor it. Be conscious that you're rewarding yourself—trust me, you'll enjoy it more! It will also help you keep track of what you're eating so you can hold yourself accountable and not go overboard.

And remember, I'm not asking you to sign a contract here. It's perfectly fine to bounce from one choice to the other. You might start out as a Convert, but wake up a year later cuddling up to an empty bag of caramel popcorn and realize you're a Realist.

No matter how you choose to maintain **Sugar Free 3**, always, *always* remember the point isn't to deprive or punish yourself, and you can reboot with another round of **SF3** anytime you need it.

CHAPTER

CHAPTER

10

THE OPENFIT ADVANTAGE

Download the Simple, Efficient, and Fun
Digital Companion to the Book

S O YOU'VE HEARD me talk about Openfit. I'll start by saying that they are my partner in **Sugar Free 3**, and now they can be yours. Openfit is a brand-new, fully integrated digital streaming platform for fitness, nutrition, and wellness. Their team has over two decades of experience creating video and digital-based healthy nutrition, weight loss, and fitness programs.

In addition to this book, we've created a streaming version of this program on the Openfit app that can be used alone or as the companion to this book, which includes exclusive content you won't find anywhere else. Not only can you get a customized 21-day meal plan and simple meal tracking, once you join you'll have instant access to my videos where I explain all the allowed foods and the ones to avoid, what to eat every day, plus educational videos on reading labels, weight loss with my good friend and registered dietitian Keri Glassman, and so much more.

You can follow the program your way—with the book or the app— but for best results I recommend you use them together. Here's a detailed breakdown of what you get. All you have to do is go to Openfit. com/**SF3** to get started.

MEAL PLANNING & TRACKING

Once you sign up and download the app, you get access to so much great content, including:

- *Step-by-step onboarding and goal setting*
- *21-day customized meal plan to help you eliminate the guesswork*
- *Automatically build your grocery list from your meal plan with only a few taps on your phone*
- *Track your meals and results*
- *Extensive food lists with every food you can imagine at your fingertips*
- *Dining out guide*
- *All the videos (more on that in a second)*

RECIPES

I've worked with the registered dietitians at Openfit and some amazing chefs to create over 80 sugar-free and delicious recipes you and your family will love. They're so good you won't believe they're sugar-free—but they are. Many are here in the book, but there are lots of exclusive ones waiting for you on the Openfit app. Most can be made in 30 minutes or less!

◆ *Plus you'll find hundreds of additional Sugar Free 3-approved recipes in the database for you to try!*

EXCLUSIVE VIDEOS

Get the complete program delivered in digital format. I'll teach you everything you need to know, and you can access the videos right from your phone. Some of the great videos include:

◆ *Allowed foods.* See all the foods you can eat.

◆ *Not Allowed foods.* Learn all the foods to avoid and why.

◆ *Reading labels.* Keri Glassman, MS, RD, CDN, teaches you steps to read a label and determine which foods are approved and not.

◆ *A day in the life.* I'll show you what to eat whether you like to cook, or will be dining out, or ordering in for every meal. I promise this program fits into your life.

◆ *Weight loss.* When you cut added sugars, you often shed excess pounds, but if weight loss is your goal you'll want to watch this video to accelerate your results.

◆ *Dining out.* My personal tips for conquering restaurants and any social situation.

◆ *Plus:* Crush your Cravings, Day 22 and Beyond, and more!

SWEET TALK DAILY VIDEOS

We all could use a little daily motivation. Just select your start date and you'll have access to my daily video filled with tips and motivation to keep you going!

EXCLUSIVE COMMUNITY FOR YOU TO JOIN

Change is always hard, and doing **Sugar Free 3** isn't easy. But you don't have to go it alone. Join me and thousands of people like you supporting each other every step of the way! We share meal ideas, recipes, food finds, we'll answer your questions, and we're here to help you overcome every challenge. Let's do this together!

WORKOUTS THAT WORK FOR YOU

Access over 300 workouts. Join a live fitness class led by certified trainers who can give you real-time feedback to help you get the most out of your workouts. Or stream results-driven on-demand programs led by world-class trainers. You'll find barre, high-intensity interval training, Pilates, yoga, cardio, strength training, running and walking classes, and special movement videos with Lauren Roxburgh designed specially for *SF3*.

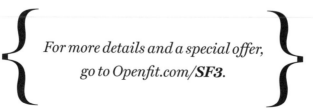

*For more details and a special offer, go to Openfit.com/**SF3**.*

APPENDIX

Tools That Help You Make
the Right Choice Every Time

The Expanded Food List

TOTALLY ALLOWED

Enjoy these foods at mealtimes or as snacks.

NSA = no sugar added

Healthy Proteins

Beef, lean (eye round, flank steak, flap steak, sirloin tip, tenderloin, top sirloin)

Beef, ground (≥ 85% lean)

Bison/buffalo

Chicken, skinless

Chicken, ground (≥ 93% lean)

Deli meat slices (NSA, nitrate- and nitrite-free)

Eggs (whole, whites, pre-boiled, cartoned, etc.)

Jerky (NSA, nitrate- and nitrite-free; all varieties)

Pork, (tenderloin, chop, top loin roast, rib chop)

Protein powder (NSA; pea, whey, hemp, etc.)

Openfit Plant-Based Protein Shake

Ostrich

Tempeh

Tofu

Turkey, skinless

Turkey, ground (≥ 93% lean)

Venison

Fish & Shellfish

Ahi

Anchovies

Chilean sea bass

Clams

Cod

Crab

Crawfish

Flounder

Haddock

Halibut

Herring

Lobster

Mackerel

Mahi-mahi

Mussels

Pollock

Oysters

Salmon (fresh, canned, or smoked)

Sardines (fresh or canned)

Scallops

Shrimp

Skate

Sole

Squid

Tilapia

Trout (fresh or smoked)

Tuna (fresh, canned, or pouched)

Whitefish

Whiting

Ceviche

Poké (NSA)

Sashimi

Sushi (wrapped in cucumber or seaweed; no rice)

Beans & Legumes

Adzuki beans

Bean pasta

Black beans

Cannellini beans

Edamame/Soybeans

Fava beans

Garbanzo beans / Chickpeas

Great northern beans

Hummus (and other NSA bean spreads)

Kidney beans

Lentils (all colors)

Lima beans

Mung beans

Navy beans

Peas (black-eyed, cow, green, etc.)

Pinto beans

Vegetables

Artichokes

Arugula

Asparagus

Beet greens

Beets

Bell pepper (all varieties)

Bok choy

Broccoli

Broccolini

Brussels sprouts

Cabbage (red, napa, Chinese, etc.)

Cactus

Carrots (all varieties)

Celery

Celery root

Chard

Collard greens

Cucumbers (all varieties)

Dandelion greens

Eggplant

Endive

Fennel

Fermented veggies (kimchi, sauerkraut, etc.)

Green beans

Hearts of palm

Jerusalem artichoke

Jicama

Kale

Kohlrabi

Leek

Lettuce (romaine, butter, etc.)

Mesclun

Mustard greens

Okra

Onions (red, white, green, etc.)

Mushrooms (oyster, porcini, portobello, etc.)

Pickles

Radicchio

Radishes/daikon

Rapini (broccoli rabe)

Rhubarb

Rutabaga

Seaweed (raw or dried)

Shallots

Snow peas

Spinach

Sprouts

String beans

Sugar snap peas

Summer squash (chayote, yellow, spagetti, etc.)

Swiss chard

Tomatillos

Tomatoes (all varieties)

Turnip

Turnip greens

Water chestnuts

Watercress

Zucchini

Unsweetened Flavor Enhancers

Allspice

Basil

Cacao powder

Cardamon

Cayenne

Chives

Cilantro

Cinnamon

Curry powder

Dill

Everything But the Bagel seasoning

Fennel

Garlic

Ginger

Horseradish

Hot sauce (NSA)

Lemon (fresh-squeezed)

Lime (fresh-squeezed)

Mint

Mustard (NSA)

Nutmeg

Nutritional Yeast

Oregano

Paprika

Parsley

Pepper

Pico de gallo (NSA)

Rosemary

Sage

Salsa (NSA; fresh, bottled, canned)

Sea salt

Seasoning blends (NSA)

Soy sauce

Spice blend (NSA)

Sriracha (NSA)

Tamari sauce

Tarragon

Thyme

Turmeric

Vinaigrette (NSA)

Vinegar (except balsamic)

Beverages

Coffee

Tea

Water (sparkling or flat; seltzer, club soda, etc.)

ALLOWED IN MODERATION

These foods are still approved, but often higher in calories,
so they can be enjoyed in moderation at every meal.

Starchy Veggies

Cassava/Yuca
Corn
Parsnips
Plantains
Potatoes, (red, white,
    Yukon, etc.)
Sweet potato
Taro
Turnips
Winter squash (acorn,
    butternut, pumpkin, etc.)
Yam

Whole Fruit

Apples
Apricots
Banana
Blackberries
Blueberries
Cherries
Figs
Grapefruit
Grapes
Guava
Jackfruit
Kiwifruit
Mango
Melon (cantaloupe,
    honeydew, etc.)
Nectarine
Orange
Papaya
Passion fruit
Peach
Pear
Pineapple
Plum
Pluot
Pomegranate
Raspberries
Strawberries
Tangerine

Unrefined Whole Grains

Amaranth
Barley (except pearled)
Bread (NSA, 100% whole-
    grain or sprouted)
Buckwheat
Bulgur
Corn meal
Crackers (NSA, 100%
    whole-grain or
    sprouted)
Farro
Freekeh
Millet
Oats/Oatmeal (NSA)
Popcorn (NSA, no trans
    fat)
Pasta (NSA, 100% whole-
    grain or sprouted)
Quinoa
Rice, brown
Rice, wild
Sorghum
Spelt
Teff
Wraps (NSA, 100% whole-
    grain or sprouted)

Healthy Fats

Avocado
Cacao nibs
Coconut (NSA)
Mayonnaise (NSA)
Nut & seed butters
    (NSA; almond, peanut,
    cashew, etc.)
Nuts (unsalted, all
    varieties)
Oil (extra virgin olive,
    avocado, coconut, etc.)
Olives
Pesto
Seeds (chia, flax, hemp,
    etc.)
Tahini

Dairy

Butter (ghee)
Cottage cheese (plain)
Cheese (light, full-fat;
    blue, feta, cheddar, etc.)
Cream cheese
Greek yogurt (plain)
Kefir (plain)
Milk (whole, reduced-fat,
    low-fat, skim)
Milk, plant-based (NSA;
    almond, soy, oat, etc.)
Sour cream
Vegan cheese (NSA)
Vegan yogurt (NSA)
Yogurt (plain)

Other Flavor Enhancers

Ketchup (NSA)
Marinades (NSA)
Miso
Pasta sauces (NSA)
Salad dressings (NSA)
Tapenade (NSA)

Stevia & Monk fruit

Stevia (liquid or powder)
Monk fruit (liquid or powder)

BARELY ALLOWED

These foods are sanctioned on this plan, but we recommend limiting.

High-Fat Proteins

Bacon (NSA)
Beef, fatty (T-bone, rib-eye, rib roast, prime rib, short ribs, back ribs)
Beef, ground (<85% fat)
Ham
Hot dogs
Lamb
Pork, fatty (belly, back ribs, spareribs, shoulder)
Salami
Sausage

Unhealthy Fats

Bottled dressings (NSA)
French fries
Palm oil
Potato chips
Tortilla chips

NOT ALLOWED

Avoid these ingredients and foods.

Alcohol (beer, liquor, wine)
Bagels
Brownies
Cakes
Candy (gummies, sour candies, etc.)
Candy bars
Cereals (refined grain or sugar-added)
Chocolate
Coffee creamer (sugar added)
Cookies
Croissants
Donuts
Dried fruit
Energy bars
Fried, batttered foods (fish, chicken, tempura, etc.)
Fruit juices and concentrates
Granola bars
Gravy
Gum (even sugar-free)
Honey mustard
Ice cream
Jams/Jellies/Preserves
Ketchup (sugar added)
Muffins
Pancake mixes (refined grain or sugar-added)
Pastries
Pizza/Pizza dough (refined grain or sugar-added)
Pretzels (refined grain or sugar-added)
Processed cheese spreads (sugar-added)
Refined and enriched flour products (bread, crackers, wraps, pasta, etc.)
Shaved ice

Soda (diet and regular)
Sugar-sweetened beverages (fruit-flavored drinks, energy drinks, sweetened teas, sports drinks)
Sport drinks
Yogurt (frozen or regular, sugar-added)

Sugar AKAs

Agave juice
Agave nectar
Agave syrup, all varieties
Barley malt
Beet sugar
Blackstrap molasses
Brown rice syrup
Brown sugar
Buttered syrup
Cane juice
Cane juice crystals
Cane sugar
Cane syrup
Caramel
Carob syrup
Castor sugar
Coconut sugar
Confectioner's sugar
Corn glucose syrup
Corn syrup
Corn syrup solids
Date sugar/syrup
Demerara sugar
Dextrin
Dextrose
Diastatic malt
Drimol
Ethyl maltol
Evaporated cane juice
Flo malt
Florida crystals

[NOT ALLOWED, *continued*]

Fructose
Fructose sweetener
Fruit juice
Fruit juice concentrate
Glucose
Glucose solids
Golden sugar
Golden syrup
Granular sweetener
Granulated sugar
Grape sugar
High fructose corn syrup (HFC)
Honey
Honibake
Icing sugar
Inverted sugar aka invert sugar
Isoglucose
Isomaltulose
Kona-ame
Malt syrup
Malt, all varieties
Maltodextrin
Maltose
Maple
Maple sugar
Maple syrup
Mizu-ame
Molasses
Muscovado sugar
Nulomoline
Panela sugar
Powdered sugar
Raw sugar
Refiner's syrup
Rice syrup
Sorghum syrup
Starch sweetener
Sucanat
Sucrovert
Sugar beet
Treacle or treacle sugar
Turbinado sugar
Unrefined sugar
Yellow sugar

Artificial Sweeteners

Acesulfame Potassium (ACK, Ace K, Equal Spoonful [also +aspartame], Sweet One, Sunett)

Aspartame (APM, AminoSweet [but not in US], aspartyl-phenylalanine-1-methyl ester, Equal Classic, NatraTaste Blue, NutraSweet)

Aspartame-acesulfame salt

Cyclamate (calcium cyclamate, Sucaryl)

Glycerol (glycerin, glycerine)

Glycyrrhizin (licorice)

Neotame

Saccharin (acid saccharin, Equal Saccharin, Necta Sweet, sodium saccharin, Sweet N Low, Sweet Twin)

Sucralose ([1',4,6'] trichlorogalactosucrose, trichlorosucrose, Equal Sucralose, NatraTaste Gold, Splenda)

Tagatose (Natrulose)

Sugar Alcohols

Erythritol (sugar alcohol, Zerose, ZSweet)

Hydrogenated Starch Hydrolysate (HSH) (sugar alcohol)

Isomalt (sugar alcohol, ClearCut Isomalt, Decomalt, DiabetiSweet [also contains Acesulfame-K], hydrogenated isomaltulose, isomaltitol)

Lactitol (sugar alcohol)

Maltitol (sugar alcohol, maltitol syrup, maltitol powder, hydrogenated high maltose content glucose syrup, hydrogenated maltose, Lesys, MaltiSweet [hard to find online to buy], SweetPearl)

Mannitol (sugar alcohol)

Polydextrose (sugar alcohol; derived from glucose and sorbitol)

Sorbitol (sugar alcohol, D-glucitol, D-glucitol syrup)

Xylitol (sugar alcohol, Smart Sweet, Xylipure, Xylosweet)

The Sugar Free 3– Approved Brands

Now that you've learned foods that are approved and how to read a nutrition label and ingredients list in order to spot added sugars, you'll be able to avoid them with ease. To make life even easier, I collected this list of brands that have no added sugars. While by no means comprehensive, it makes for a quick-and-easy shopper's guide. With this many choices, you'll never go hungry on **Sugar Free 3.**

MILKS

When it comes to cow or goat milk, I recommend low-fat, reduced-fat, or whole milk.

Almond Milk

365 Everyday Value Organic Almondmilk Unsweetened

Almond Breeze Unsweetened Almond Milk

Califia Farms Unsweetened Almond Milk

Califia Farms Unsweetened Vanilla Almond Milk

Silk Unsweetened Almond Milk

Silk Unsweetened Vanilla Almond Milk

Silk Organic Unsweetened Almond Milk

Silk Organic Unsweetened Vanilla Almond Milk

Silk Unsweetened Almond Coconut Blend

Soy Milk

Silk Organic Unsweetened Soy Milk

365 Everyday Value Organic Unsweetened Soy Milk

Unsweetened Edensoy, Organic

Wildwood Organic Soy Milk, Unsweetened

Oat Milk

Califia Farms Unsweetened Oat Milk

Califia Farms Unsweetened Übermilk

Califia Farms Unsweetened Vanilla Übermilk

Dream Oat Beverage, Unsweetened

Oatly Oat Milk

Oatly Low-Fat Oat Milk

Silk Oat Yeah The Plain One Oat Milk

Coconut Milk

365 Everyday Value Organic Unsweetened Original Coconut Milk Beverage

Califia Farms Go Coconuts Coconut Milk

Coconut Dream Unsweetened Coconut Drink

Silk Unsweetened Coconut Milk

Cashew Milk

Califia Farms Organic Cashew Homestyle Nutmilk

Silk Unsweetened Cashew Milk

YOGURT

Always read the nutrition label—don't judge a yogurt by its cover. Many yogurts have added sugars or artificial sweeteners. Same goes for "dairy-free" yogurts made from soy, almond milk, soy milk, oat milk, or coconut.

Regular Yogurts

Dannon Lowfat Plain

Dannon Whole Milk Plain

Green Valley Organic Plain Lowfat Yogurt

Stonyfield Organic Low Fat Plain

Stonyfield Organic Whole Milk Plain

365 Everyday Value Organic Lowfat Yogurt

365 Everyday Value Organic Whole Milk Yogurt

Greek Yogurts

365 Everyday Value Organic Greek Whole Milk Yogurt, Plain

Chobani Low-Fat Plain

Fage Total 2% Plain

Fage Total 4% Plain

Fage Total Whole Plain

The Greek Gods Traditional Plain

Kalona Supernatural Organic Greek Yogurt

Maple Hill Organic Greek Yogurt Plain

Green Valley Greek Plain Yogurt 2%

Green Valley Greek Plain Yogurt Whole Milk

Stonyfield Organic Whole Milk Greek Plain

Voskos Original Plain

Wallaby Organic Aussie Greek

Whole Milk Plain

Whole Foods 365 Organic Plain Greek Lowfat Yogurt

Whole Foods 365 Organic Plain Greek Whole Milk Yogurt

Icelandic Yogurt

Icelandic Provisions Traditional Skyr Plain

Siggi's No Added Sugar Banana & Cinnamon

Siggi's No Added Sugar Raspberry & Apple—this new line is sweetened with the fruit itself

Trader Joe's Icelandic Plain

Cream Top Yogurt

Brown Cow Whole Milk Plain

Kalona Supernatural Organic Lowfat Plain

Goat's Milk Yogurt

Redwood Hill Farm Traditional Plain

Kefir

365 Everyday Value Kefir Cultured Whole Milk, Plain

Green Valley Plain Lowfat Kefir

Green Valley Plain Whole Milk Kefir

Lifeway Lowfat Organic Plain Unsweetened

Lifeway Whole Milk Organic Plain Unsweetened

Maple Hill Plain Unsweetened

Redwood Hill Farm Plain

Siggi's Filmjölk Plain

Wallaby Organic Aussie Kefir Lowfat Plain

CEREALS

Cold Cereals

365 Everyday Value Wheat Squares

Arrowhead Mills Bulgur Wheat

Arrowhead Mills Puffed Barley

Arrowhead Mills Puffed Corn

Arrowhead Mills Puffed Kamut

Arrowhead Mills Puffed Millet

Barbara's Shredded Wheat

Ezekiel 4:9 Sprouted Whole Grain
Cereal Original

Ezekiel 4:9 Sprouted Whole Grain
Cereal Golden Flax

Post Shredded Wheat Original
Spoon Size

Post Shredded Wheat Big Biscuit

Quaker Puffed Wheat

Hot Cereals

365 Everyday Value Organic Instant
Oatmeal Original

365 Everyday Value Organic Quick Cook
Steel Cut Oats

Arrowhead Mills Organic Gluten Free
Rice and Shine Hot Cereal

Arrowhead Mills Steel Cut Oats
Hot Cereal

Quaker Oats Old Fashioned & Quick
Oats

Quaker Oats Steel Cut

McCann's Irish Oatmeal

Bob's Red Mill Old-Fashioned Oats

Purely Elizabeth—Original Superfood
Oatmeal

BREADS

Just because you see the words
wheat, enriched, or *sprouted* doesn't
mean it's **SF3**-approved. Look for
the words *whole wheat* or *whole
grain*. And watch out for sugars in
the ingredients list! Search for the
breads below, often found in your
refrigerator or freezer aisle.

Sliced Bread

Ezekiel 4:9 Sprouted Whole Grain Bread

Ezekiel 4:9 Low-Sodium Sprouted
Whole Grain Bread

Ezekiel 4:9 Flax Sprouted Whole Grain
Bread

Manna Organics Sunseed Bread

Manna Organics Millet Rice

Manna Organics Multigrain

Manna Organics Whole Rye

Wraps, Pita, and Tortillas

Ezekiel 4:9 Whole Grain Pocket Bread

Ezekiel 4:9 Sprouted Whole Grain Tortillas

English Muffins

Ezekiel 4:9 7 Sprouted Grain
English Muffins

Ezekiel 4:9 Sprouted Grain Flax
English Muffins

Ezekiel 4:9 Sprouted Whole Grain
English Muffins

PROCESSED MEAT

There's often sugar and other bad stuff hiding in your meat, so look for these instead.

Deli Section

365 Everyday Value Oven-Roasted Turkey Breast Deli Slices, 98% Lean

Applegate Organic Roasted Turkey Breast

Applegate Natural Herb Turkey Breast

Applegate Natural Roast Beef

Applegate Natural Roasted Turkey Breast

Applegate Natural Smoked Turkey Breast

Boar's Head 1st Cut Cooked Corned Beef Brisket

Boar's Head All Natural Cap-Off Top Round Oven Roasted Beef

Boar's Head Deluxe Low-Sodium Roasted Beef— Cap-Off Top Round

Bacon and Sausages

Applegate Organics Sweet Italian

Pederson's No Sugar Chorizo Ground Sausage

Pederson's No Sugar Italian Ground Sausage

Trader Joe's No Sugar Dry Rubbed Bacon

CONDIMENTS

Ketchup

It's nearly impossible to find ketchup without some form of added sugar. Use our **Sugar Free 3** Ketchup recipe on page 136.

Mayonnaise

Primal Kitchen Mayo with Avocado Oil

Sir Kensington

Mustard

365 Everyday Value Organic German Mustard

365 Everyday Value Organic Yellow Mustard

Annie's Organic Yellow Mustard

French's Deli Spicy Brown Mustard

OrganicVille Dijon Mustard No Added Sugar

Hot Sauce

Frank's Red Hot Hot Sauce

Trader Joe's Yuzu Hot Sauce

Vinegars

Try vinegars as condiments—wine vinegars, apple cider vinegar, white vinegar—to add flavor without sugar. Just avoid balsamic.

RICE AND PASTA

Rice

Look for brown rice—dry or precooked—any brand.

Birds Eye Riced Cauliflower

Carolina Brown Rice, Whole Grain

Green Giant Caulifower Rice

Minute Brown Rice, Whole Grain

Trader Joe's Cauliflower Rice

Uncle Ben's Ready Rice, Whole Grain

Pasta

Any whole grain or whole wheat pasta, even bean pasta.

365 Everyday Value Whole Grain Pasta

Banza Chickpea Pasta

Barilla Whole Grain Angel Hair

Barilla Whole Grain Linguini

Barilla Whole Grain Spaghetti

Barilla Whole Grain Thin Spaghetti

Explore Black Bean Pastas

Ezekiel 4:9 Sprouted Whole Grain Elbow Pasta

Ezekiel 4:9 Sprouted Whole Grain Fettuccine

Ezekiel 4:9 Sprouted Whole Grain Penne Pasta

Ezekiel 4:9 Sprouted Whole Grain Spaghetti

Palmini Hearts of Palm Pasta

Racconto 8 Whole Grain Spaghetti

Racconto 8 Whole Grain Capellini

Ronzoni Healthy Harvest Lasagna

Ronzoni Healthy Harvest Linguini

Ronzoni Healthy Harvest Penne

Ronzoni Healthy Harvest Rotini

Ronzoni Healthy Harvest Ancient Grains Thin Spaghetti

Ronzoni Healthy Harvest Ancient Grains Penne

Sam Mills Pasta d'oro Corn Pasta

Shiritaki Rice and Pasta

Spotlight on... Alternative Pastas

Enter your local market and you may find veggie pasta spirals from zucchini to sweet potato to butternut squash. You may also see chickpea or black bean pasta and even Palmini pasta in a can made from hearts of palm.

Add **SF3** Marinara, spinach, garlic, and oil, or however you love to eat pasta.

And for those who are interested, the word "shirataki" translates to "white waterfall" in Japanese, which mimics the actual look of these noodles, which are made from the konjac plant. They're thin and translucent. You can find them packaged dry or "wet" (packaged in liquid). In fact, the thing that makes shirataki noodles unique is the fact that they're mostly water—about 97% water, in fact! Depending on the brand, you'll see anywhere from 0 to 15 calories in the entire package. If you're purchasing the wet variety, you'll want to rinse them first and, depending on the packaging's instructions, parboil them before using in recipes. The dry version will have a more pasta-like consistency. Eat them in a stir-fry or a shrimp salad.

NUT BUTTERS

Peanut Butters

Santa Cruz

Maranatha Peanut Butter

Teddie All Natural Peanut Butter

Smucker's Natural Crunchy or Creamy
(not the reduced-fat)

Crazy Richard's

Almond Butters

Maranatha

Justin's Classic Almond Butter

365 Everyday Value Almond Butter

365 Everyday Value Organic Creamy
Almond Butter, Unsweetened &
No Salt

SEASONINGS

Most spices and seasonings are sugar-free, but always check the ingredients. A big hit among those who first tried **Sugar Free 3** was Everything But the Bagel seasoning from Trader Joe's.

TJ's South African Smoke Seasoning

TJ's 21 Seasoning Salute

TJ's Mushroom and Company
Multipurpose Umami Seasoning Blend

TJ's Chile Lime Seasoning Blend

TJ's Dukkah

PASTA SAUCE

Every tomato sauce has sugar, thanks to the natural sugars in the tomatoes. But the following popular brands have no sugar added. Mangia!

Classico Riserva Tomato Marinara

Classico Riserva Roasted Garlic

Classico Riserva Triple Olive Puttanesca

Classico Riserva Eggplant & Artichoke

Dell'Amore Romana

Dell'Amore Original Recipe

Dell'Amore Sweet Basil and Garlic

Dell'Amore Spicy Recipe

De Cecco Sugo alle Olive

De Cecco Sugo al Basilico

De Cecco Sugo al Pomodoro

De Cecco Sugo Delizie di Verdure

De Cecco Pesto alla Genovese

De Cecco Ragù alla Bolognese

Rao's Artichoke Sauce

Rao's Arrabbiata Sauce

Rao's 4 Cheese Sauce

Rao's Garden Vegetable Sauce

Rao's Homemade Marinara Sauce

Rao's Puttanesca Sauce

Rao's Roasted Eggplant Sauce

Rao's Roasted Garlic Sauce

Rao's Tomato Basil Sauce

SOUPS

My grandma never put sugar in her chicken soup. But many brands do. You're safe with these.

Amy's Organic Black Bean Vegetable Soup

Amy's Organic Lentil Vegetable Soup

Amy's Organic Lentil Soup

Amy's Organic Mushroom Bisque with Porcini

Amy's Organic Quinoa, Kale & Red Lentil

Amy's Organic Split Pea Soup

Amy's Organic Summer Corn & Vegetable Soup

Amy's Organic Vegan Chunky Tomato Bisque

Campbell's Ready to Serve Low Sodium Chicken Broth

Rao's Tomato Basil Soup

SMARTER SNACKS

Bars

Most nutrition and protein bars belong behind bars: They're filled with sugar and artificial sweeteners. I like an RxBar when I've got somewhere to be and no time to prepare.

Crackers

Mary's Gone Crackers—all flavors

GG Crackers

Triscuits

Tortilla Chips

Garden of Eatin' Baked Blue Chips

Garden of Eatin' Baked Yellow Chips

Garden of Eatin' Sunny Blues

Garden of Eatin' Veggie Chips

Way Better Multi-Grain

Way Better Black Bean

Way Better Blue Corn

Way Better Ginger Sweet Potato

Way Better No Salt Naked Blues

Wise White Restaurant Style Tortillas

Veggie or Legume-Based Chips

Enjoy Life Grab & Go Lentil Chips Sea Salt

Enjoy Life Grab & Go Lentil Chips Garlic & Parmesan

Enjoy Life Grab & Go Lentil Chips Margherita Pizza

Enjoy Life Grab & Go Lentil Chips Thai Chili Lime

Rhythm Organic Cauliflower Bites

Rhythm Organic Beet Chips

Rhythm Organic Carrot Sticks

Rhythm Organic Kale Chips

Simply 7 Lentil Chips Sea Salt

Simply 7 Quinoa Chips Sea Salt

Popcorn

Boom Chicka Pop Sea Salt

Good Health Half Naked Hint of Olive Oil

Good Health Half Naked Organic Sea Salt

My Favorite Smarter Snacks

Green apple with cinnamon • Green apple with almond butter

Mary's Gone Crackers with hummus • Cucumber with guacamole

Air-popped popcorn • Biltong (no sugar added)

Go Lite Himalayan Salt

SkinnyPop Original

SkinnyPop Sea Salt & Pepper

Smartfood Delight Sea Salt

Note: Popcorners Salt of the Earth chips are also sugar-free.

Bean Snacks

Bada Bean Bada Boom Sea Salt

Brami Lupini Beans Sea Salt

Brami Chili Lime

Brami Hot Chili Pepper

Enlightened Roasted Broad Bean Crisps

Cruncha ma-me Dried Edamane

DIPS AND SPREADS

Salsa

365 Everyday Value Salsa, Medium Thick & Chunky

Amy's Salsa Mild, Medium, and Black Bean & Corn

Muir Glen Organic Salsas, Mild, Medium, Garlic Cilantro, Black Bean, and Corn

Tostitos Chunky Salsa Mild, Medium, and Hot

Trader Joe's Extra Hot Ghost Pepper Salsa

Trader Joe's Homestyle Salsa Especial Medium

Trader Joe's Roasted Tomatillo Salsa

Wise Salsa Mild and Medium

Guacamole

Fresh is best, but...

Cabo Fresh Guacamole Authentic

Cabo Fresh Guacamole Fiesta

Sabra Guacamole

Sabra Guacamole with Lime

Wholly Guacamole—all varieties

Hummus, regular or organic

Athenos Original Hummus, all varieties

Cedar's Classic Original Hommus

Cedar's Everything Hommus

Cedar's Sundried Tomato & Basil Hommus

Cedar's Garlic Lovers Hommus

Cedar's Roasted Red Pepper Hommus

Cedar's Roasted Eggplant Hommus

Cedar's Artichoke Spinach Hommus

Sabra Basil Pesto Hummus

Sabra Jalepeño Hummus

Sabra Classic Hummus

Sabra Lemon Twist Hummus

Sabra Roasted Garlic Hummus

Trader Joe's Organic Spicy Avocado Hummus

Trader Joe's Roasted Garlic Hummus

Tribe Classic Hummus

Tribe Mediterranean Style

Tribe Roasted Garlic

Tribe Roasted Red Pepper

CRUSTS

365 Everyday Value Cauliflower Pizza Crust

Outer Aisle Plantpower Pizza Crusts and Sandwich Thins

Cali'Flour Foods Pizza Crust

Trader Joe's Broccoli & Kale Pizza Crust

Trader Joe's Cauliflower Pizza Crust

BEVERAGES

Bubly Sparkling Water

LaCroix

Perrier Sparkling Mineral Water

Poland Spring Sparkling

Polar Seltzer, all flavors

Vintage Seltzer

Waterloo Sparkling Water

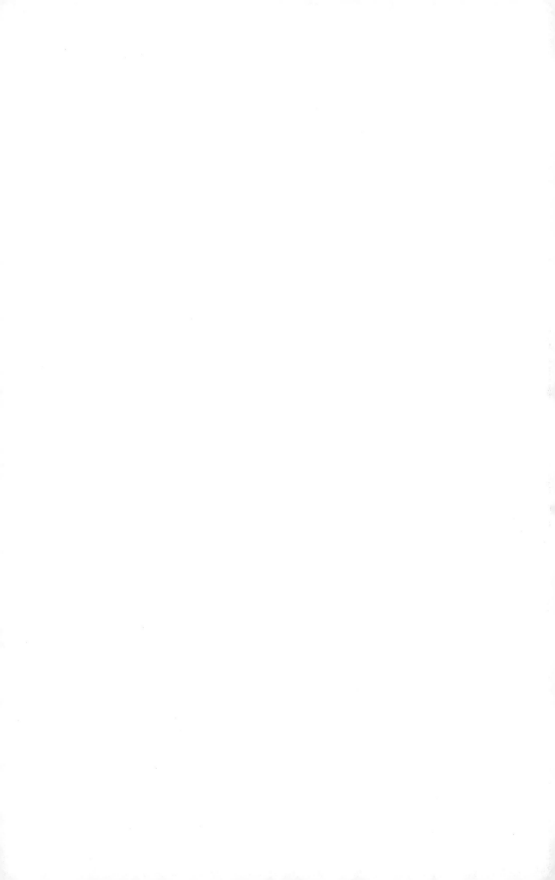

SUGAR TRACKER

Your 7-Day Personal Journal

DAY 1

DATE:

WEIGHT:

BREAKFAST:

LUNCH:

DINNER:

SNACKS:

WATER (IN OUNCES):

MINDFUL INDULGENCE:

I EXERCISED:

TODAY I FEEL:

DAY 2

DATE:

WEIGHT:

BREAKFAST:

LUNCH:

DINNER:

SNACKS:

WATER (IN OUNCES):

MINDFUL INDULGENCE:

I EXERCISED:

TODAY I FEEL:

DAY 3

DATE:

WEIGHT:

BREAKFAST:

LUNCH:

DINNER:

SNACKS:

WATER (IN OUNCES):

MINDFUL INDULGENCE:

I EXERCISED:

TODAY I FEEL:

DAY 4

DATE:

WEIGHT:

BREAKFAST:

LUNCH:

DINNER:

SNACKS:

WATER (IN OUNCES):

MINDFUL INDULGENCE:

I EXERCISED:

TODAY I FEEL:

DAY 5

DATE:

WEIGHT:

BREAKFAST:

LUNCH:

DINNER:

SNACKS:

WATER (IN OUNCES):

MINDFUL INDULGENCE:

I EXERCISED:

TODAY I FEEL:

DAY 6

DATE:

WEIGHT:

BREAKFAST:

LUNCH:

DINNER:

SNACKS:

WATER (IN OUNCES):

MINDFUL INDULGENCE:

I EXERCISED:

TODAY I FEEL:

DAY 7

DATE:

WEIGHT:

BREAKFAST:

LUNCH:

DINNER:

SNACKS:

WATER (IN OUNCES):

MINDFUL INDULGENCE:

I EXERCISED:

TODAY I FEEL:

ACKNOWLEDGMENTS

Teamwork Makes the Dream Work!

SUGAR FREE 3 would not have been possible without a legion of people who are driven by the purpose of empowering others to adopt healthier lifestyles. Chief among them, my talented, tireless (and also super-fun!) **SF3** development partners Lara Ross, Allie Eichner, and Jonathan Rivera. Thank you for caring as deeply as I do about making this project the absolute best it could be—and for keeping me energized with a never-ending supply of healthy snacks. A special shoutout is owed to Denis Faye, MS, Openfit's executive director of nutrition, and his colleagues Andrea Giancoli, MPH, RD, Kirsten Morningstar, and Krista Maguire, RD, CSSD. Line by line, they ensured every word was nutritionally bulletproof.

Galvanized Media, I'm grateful. Founder David Zinczenko is a BFF, brother from another mother, and inspiring mentor all in one. He knows a thing or two (thousand) about how to write books that help people take control of their health, and his guidance was so valuable. There isn't enough praise on the planet for my lead editor, Michael Freidson, who helped me pull it all together with the most even, calm temperament. I attribute his impressively stable mood to the fact that he managed to kick sugary junk food even pre–**Sugar Free 3**! Design director Joe Heroun nailed the vision, cover to cover, and designer Laura White executed it flawlessly (while juggling a million little pieces). Michael Martin and Rebecca Maines made sure the words made sense.

I'm a wellness journalist and editor, not a credentialed expert. That's why I was so lucky to have Keri Glassman, MS, RD, CDN; Max Lugavere, author of *Genius Foods*; my personal dermatologist, Dr. Whitney Bowe; movement expert Lauren Roxburgh; and bio-alchemist Michelle Gagnon contribute their enlightening insights.

A big "woo-hoo!" to the trial groups who did the first rounds of **Sugar Free 3**. You are all heroes for committing, and your feedback will help every single person reading these pages. Congrats on your success!

And finally, I thank you, the reader, for buying this book. Your trust is a privilege. I'll earn it with results.

—Michele

Index

Note: Page numbers in italics indicate recipes.

B

D

H

"health halo" trick labels, 27–30
  about: overview of, 27
  "enriched" label, 29
  "gluten-free" label, 28
  "high energy" label, 29–30
  "natural" label, 27
  "organic" label, 28
  "wheat" or "multigrain" labels, 29
heart disease, sugar and, xvii, 33
Herb Puree, *132*
herbs and spices, 73–74, 190
"high energy" label, 29–30
high fructose corn syrup (HFCS).
    See also sugar AKAs
    historical perspective, 21
    products with, 92, 98, 102
    reading food labels for, 40, 96, 97
hot sauce (NSA), 72

I

inflammation, reducing, 5–6
ingredients, grocery list and shopping
    for, 46–48. *See also* Allowed
    foods; Not Allowed foods;
    specific ingredients
intermittent fasting, 106
inviting others to join, xxi–xxii
Italian restaurant food, 172
"itol" words on labels, 105

J

Japanese restaurant food, 174–75
iournaling, tracking progress, 52, 163,
    194, 206
Juicy Turkey Burgers with Avocado &
    Turkey Bacon, *125*

K

kale. *See* greens, leafy
ketchup, 92, 108, 136
kitchen
    deciding how to do food, 44
    preparing for **SF3**, 44

L

labels. *See* food labels
Lamb, 73, 95
lettuce wraps
    Easy Chicken Club Lettuce Wraps,
      155
    Vietnamese Turkey Lettuce Wraps
      with Cucumber-Peanut Relish,
      151
libido, hotter sex and, 12–13
Like to Cook meal plan. *See* meal plan,
    Like to Cook
Lugavere, Max, viii, 10, 14, 19, 61, 160,
    186
lunch
    about: Don't Cook meal plan, 158;
      fast and easy (12 minutes or less!),
      150–55; Like to Cook meal plan
      recipes, 121–27; meal-planning
      ideas, 49; planning, 45–46,
      49–50, 207; Willing to Cook meal
      plan recipes, 145, 150–55
    BLT Sweet Potato Toast, *127*
    Chicken Caesar Salad with
      Pumpkin Seeds, *122*
    Easy Chicken Club Lettuce Wraps,
      155
    Greek Chopped Salad, *121*
    Juicy Turkey Burgers with Avocado
      & Turkey Bacon, *125*
    Mediterranean Platter with Pickled
      Veggies and Tahini Drizzle, *154*

Q

R

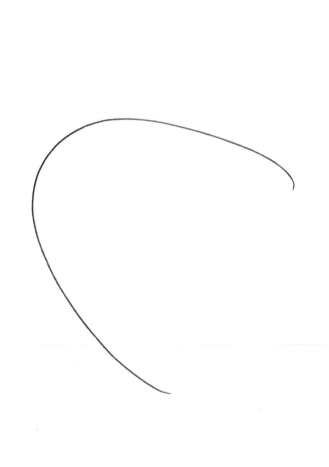